# Keeping A Breast Or Two

## A
## BREAST MAINTENANCE
## GUIDE

*By*

*Pat Sheffield*
*Medical Missionary*

The publisher assumes full responsibility for the accuracy of all information and quotations as cited in this book.

**Anchor Publishing**
Camden, Tennessee

# DEDICATION

This book is dedicated to every woman with a medical problem. Christ is asking *"Wilt thou be made whole?"* (John 5:6). It is our prayer that, by faith, she will accept the Great Physician's invitation for spiritual healing and physical restoration.

*"There is life and health in doing;
There is pleasure in pursuing;
Doing then, is health accruing;
Do Something!"*

# CONTENTS

# ACKNOWLEDGEMENTS

In the composition of any book one is
dependent, at least in part,
on the input of others.
To present a guide, as all-inclusive as possible,
different sources were used as a basis
for information flow.

# MAJOR CONTRIBUTORS

King James Version Holy Bible
Inspired Writings of Ellen G. White, a prolific writer
*(denoted by indented, italic/bold quotes and*
*book reference )*

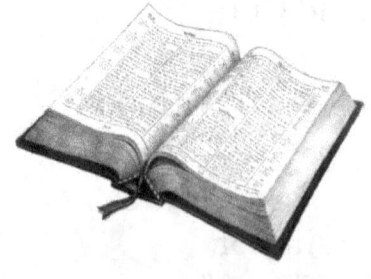

*This Owner Manual*
*belongs to:*

_____

*From*

_____

*Date*

_____

# LIFE IS A
# MAINTENANCE PROGRAM
## *AND YOU ARE THE*

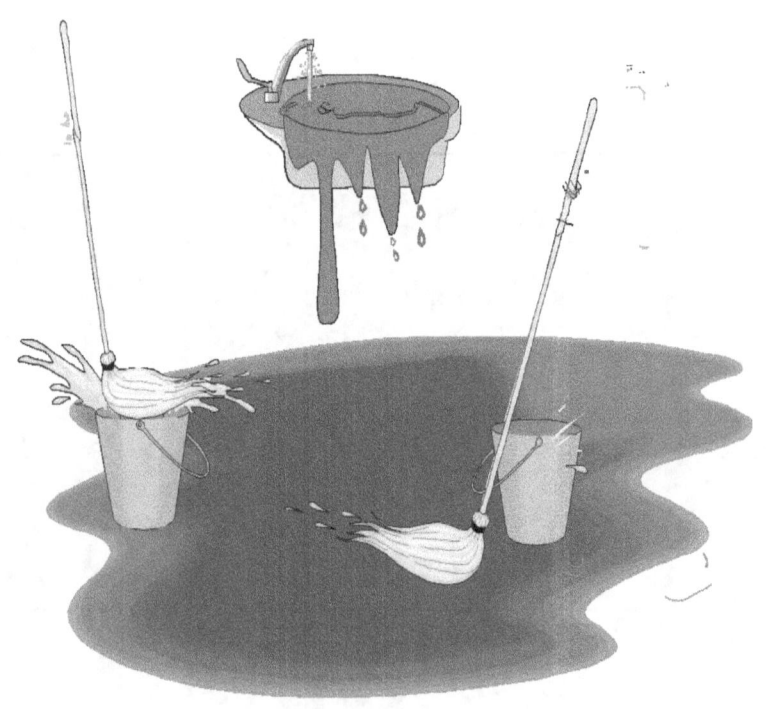

## *Breast-Maid!*

# PREFACE

In life, there are many choices that challenge us to do or not to do. Our decisions, we hope, provide the answers and comfort. Over the years, women with breast cancer have been and are still being challenged. Today, more women, young and old, face new challenges related to this lethal disease.

*"Keeping A-Breast or Two"* addresses those challenges and recognizes the importance of sharing information to help women deal with these difficulties. This handy guide was compiled to assist women with their breast-filled questions. You will discover informative, practical, to–the-point information in these pages --- including a *"how to"* section, detailing a *"health"* plan. Consider this your own personal handbook for breast support.

Since breast cancer has no boundaries now, and has reached across the globe into other countries, our approach allows this global communique to reach all classes of society, by the exchange of "healthful and helpful" tools.

As an encouragement to readers, this timely and comforting supplement, comes as a health companion, to have with you always.

Once you've finished reading this special illustrative health-bearing gift, we invite you to share it with family, friends, neighbors, and strangers. It's one of the best ways to ensure that all keep abreast, too!

# HOW TO USE THIS BOOK

If a publication is produced without a purpose then it shouldn't be printed. This manual is prepared with a purpose, and that purpose is to educate women, young and old, on how to gain victory over the besetting challenges of breast disease — all of them!

Normally, a product or service comes with a manual which provides instructions and a limited warranty. As for the breasts, they come with a complete manual, too -- namely the Holy Bible. Inspired by the Creator-Manufacturer, this Book of all books contain instructions (laws), lifetime warranties (promises), factory authorized repair and service (help), to correct any defects (sickness/disease), at no costs (plan of salvation).

Inside this manual, in scope and content, unfolds the operational layout for female breasts, detailing their inner and outer most requirements. The layout is as follows:

**Chapter 1: "Breasts Assured!"** provides structural and functional information on female breasts. With a seasonal comparison, this chapter profiles the breasts in four stages of a woman's life: infancy/childhood, youth/adolescent, adulthood, and senior adulthood.

**Chapter 2: "Got Breast Disease?"** opens with my perspective of breast disease followed by a statistical view of breast cancer, not only in the United States but globally. Additionally, profiled are the various types, stages, symptoms, as well as short descriptions of these medical conditions.

**Chapter 3: "Cause for Concern"** highlights the risk factors that wreak havoc on the female body, which in turns affect the breasts. Plainly, the causes have been searched out and outlined.

**Chapter 4: "The Big Cover-up"** uncovers additional "factors" that are utilized in day-to-day living. By design and deception, the dangers are covered up but this section brings them out of the closet.

**Chapter 5: "Remove the Cause... Not the Breasts"** section examines women's decisions that accompany the diagnosis of breast disease (cancer) and surveys the medical procedures and practices in today's society. In light of this, indispensable knowledge is presented in this section to dispel the clouds and bring reassuring answers of hope to women's lives.

**Chapter 6: "Breast Care: Prevention and Cure"** builds upon the preceding chapters by supplying women with methods and tips of taking more responsibility for their own breasts.. The chapter provides different approaches, techniques, suggestions and points of view to avoid breasts' mishaps and breakdowns or the need for major repair.

**Chapter 7:** Last but not least, **"Not By Prescription"** is packed with useful information and provides resources for launching your body into a new healthier lifestyle, with a practical health plan to follow.

Additionally, to help you understand the medical jargon used for breast cancer or other breast disorders, a glossary of medical terms has been provided in the back of this book along with "The Write Things" section to record questions, answers, instructions, suggestions that may arise.

As you warm up to the information in this book, think about building a healthier lifestyle – daily. Many women start out looking for the right answers to avoid or fix this major public health threat of breast cancer. However, what has been offered does not prove to remedy their problem. Depending on what you are seeking and what works for you, referring back to this book again and again could be the key. Each time you might see something different, depending on what you're experiencing or your level of commitment. Remember, only you can decide what to try to help you achieve healthy breasts.

More importantly, women – young and old -- to avoid future breast problems consult the User Manual (Holy Bible). It is tailor-made just for you!

# Chapter 1

## *Breasts Assured!*

*Nourishing. Life giving. Monumental to life.*

Your Breasts. A Guide. No matter which way you turn, to the right or the left, they are there. The majority of women, young and old, have a distant relationship with them. Their arrival can be startling. They can be a jolt for some at first, requiring some getting use to. There should be an ongoing commitment with them. Even learning to appreciate them requires extra effort.

The breasts are the most visible signs of womanliness. At inception, the breasts undergo changes that prepare the girl to go from infancy to womanhood. In order to understand these changes and adjustments, it helps to have a basic knowledge of their anatomy and physiology. To address some females' unfamiliarity with the breasts, we'll steer you through its structural and functional features. If you already know, just consider it a refresher course.

With the scope of the breasts vividly in mind and given that they change significantly from infancy to senior adulthood, becoming acquainted with their particular characteristics not only renders them more meaningful, but contributes to a richer understanding and appreciation of them as a whole. In addition, because of the existing differences of women, it would be a giant step towards breast awareness for us to understand the "ins and outs" of the breast in their truest sense. The following Scripture reflects on the Creator's design of female breasts, *"Thy two breasts are like two young roes that are twins,.."* (Song of Solomon 4:5).

Unmistakably, He created two!

Any explanation of the development of the breasts should always begin with a description of its fundamental unit of structure — the cell. The structural basis of all parts of the human body is the cell. All the cells throughout the body are fundamentally similar in structure and function. However, their appearance varies as they become specialized to perform their functions. Combined, they form tissues of many diverse shapes and purposes. Each cell is a minute portion of living matter separated from the other cells, the cell membrane. Each cell has its own center of activity, the nucleus. Cells are arranged into groups to form tissues and organs as the heart or the breasts. The manner of their organization and the specialized nature of the cells determine the function that the organ or the tissue can and will perform.

The breasts are an integral part of the female reproductive system. They are different by design and vary in size and shape --small, medium, large, and very large. One size does not fit all. One can better understand how the breasts work if she knows how it is constructed.

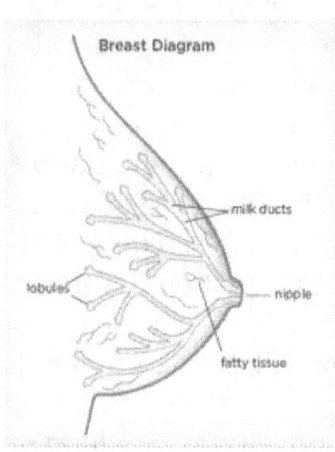

Breast Diagram

milk ducts

lobules

nipple

fatty tissue

Structurally, the breasts are accented by connective tissues, blood vessels, fat, and lymphatic channels. These components are in contact with the nipple, glands, lobes, milk ducts, and lymph nodes. Each breast is divided into loves, which are secreting glands – subdivided into several lobules (ducts). Each lobule has a small duct or passageway that unites with others to form a large duct   for each lobe, and each large duct having a minute opening at the nipple.

Securely covered by a coat of fat, the breasts thrive in a protective and insulated environment. The connective tissues bind the breasts together; attaching to the female chest wall – a kind of internal bra. The nipple is surrounded by a pigmented area called the areola in which there are many small elevations known as glands or tubercles.

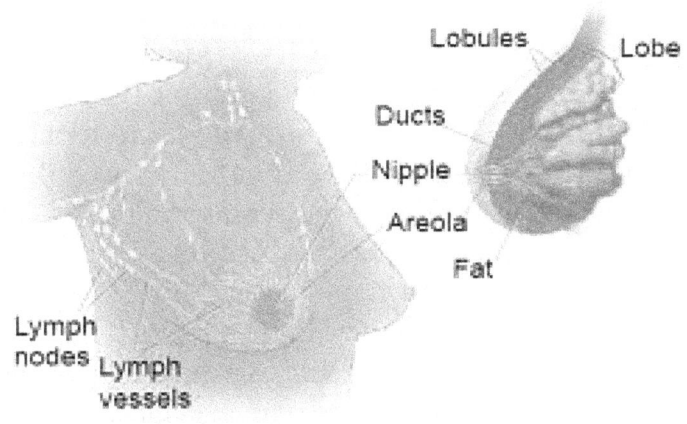

Functionally, the lobes produce the milk -- the ducts (tubes) carry milk to the nipple. The lymphatics, sometimes known as breast filters, remove fluids, draining into lymph nodes (size of kidney bean or smaller) -- playing a key role in the body's defenses against infection. All together, they play a significant part in the anatomy and physiology of the breasts.

There's a saying that "Nature is the garments of God; Scriptures are the thoughts of God." Manifestly, nature is God's thoughts made visible. *"For thou, LORD, hast made me glad through thy work: I will triumph in the works of thy* hands. *O LORD, how great are thy works! [and] thy thoughts are very deep."* (Psalms 92:4-5). Thus, the varieties of nature are adapted to the varieties of the human mind.

In our explanation of the breasts, we will compare them using nature, namely seasons — spring, summer, autumn and winter. Webster's 1828 dictionary defines *Season* as 1. A fit or suitable time; the convenient time; the usual or appointed time; 2. One of the four divisions of the year, spring, summer, autumn, winter. Using these definitions, in like fashion, the breasts duplicate the seasons as follows: 1). They constantly are changing. 2). They grow more in the first part of life than in the last part of it. 3). They act as physical markers for females, transitioning from one stage of life to another. 4). Each stage, infancy/childhood, youth/adolescent, adulthood and senior adulthood-- has its own distinctive characteristics, each emphasizes certain aspects of development, each makes unique changes, and each represents a different view of the breasts.

King Solomon declares in Ecclesiastes 3:11, *"To everything there is a <u>season</u>, and to every purpose under the heavens."* Therefore, to paint you a complete picture of the breasts, we highlight their ever-varying scenes from a seasonal view. Chronologically, we breakdown each stage of life and bring to light the activities of the breasts — in season and out of season.

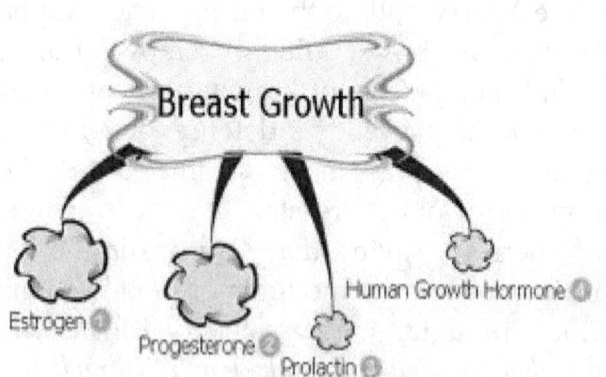

# *Spring*
# INFANCY/CHILDHOOD STAGE

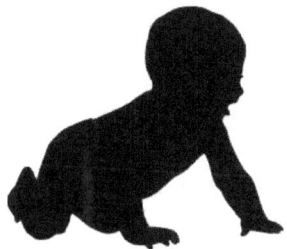 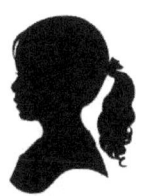

**WHAT'S GOING ON:** The baby has arrived — so has Spring! The earth has thrown off her white shroud, and nature is waking to life as spoken of in Job 38:27; *"To satisfy the <u>desolate [ground]</u> and waste, and cause the <u>bud </u>of the tender herb to spring forth?"*

In infancy, the breasts make subtle "baby steps." The breasts are undeveloped and hidden in the tiny body of the newborn, going through many changes-- just waiting it out. During the first few months, no dramatic growth is seen. However, this season of inactivity draws attention to the dawn of development signaled by visible nipples and tiny gland tissue. There's "no action" outwardly, but there is plenty inward activity going on as the breasts grow.

After relaxing for years during infancy, in childhood, the breasts are still growing inwardly, and not significantly outwardly. If some physical shifts and changes occur, the young girl generally will be inquisitive to learn things about her body. The breasts may be an "on and off" instinct in the thoughts of young girls, however, they may not be overly important to them in this stage. In the same fashion as spring prompts that it's time "to vegetate and rise out of the ground, and the seedlings begin to appear, the breasts make an appearance, with a wide range of variance in development between girls.

If questions arise in regard to the things she see and touch on her body, then mothers and guardians should take the opportunity to patiently answer these little inquiries.   At this point, while dependent upon a mother or guardian, a golden opportunity lies to teach them the ABC's of the breasts.  This quote reveals that this kind of girl talk  wouldn't be too soon:

> **"It is therefore of the highest importance, that among the studies selected for childhood, physiology should occupy the first place. How few know anything about the structure and functions of their own bodies,......how to keep their bodies in a healthy condition and prevent disease"** *Counsels on Health, p. 33.*

The ideal is for mothers or guardians to keep ahead of the pace of growth of their girls, gaining enough information to be able to explain physical manifestations when they arise. With emphasis on the breasts, by knowing your own body, such a program requires continuous study and learning.

A great way to teach anatomy and physiology to the child is through nature.  To upload, the girl's mind, have her observe the flowers and their parts as an example of introducing naturally the subject and instruct as needed. Just as the flowers start their budding in spring, so are the breasts of the young girl --up and coming.   Satisfy their curiosity  within proper limits to preoccupy that ground. Lead them into the next level of the subject, as their needs indicate.   Share some of the new experiences that the breasts will bring at puberty. On the whole, these lessons will prove beneficial, allowing her to recall those principles later in life.

Some girls' breasts may start blooming between the ages of 10-12. This could be resulting from some questionable factors that need to be addressed. (See chapters 3 and 4). Or, at her own pace, breast milestones are reached. Generally, late development should not be a major concern. If there is concern, maybe this Scripture will put your mind at rest: *"We have a little sister, and **she hath no breasts**:.." (Song* of Solomon 8:8).

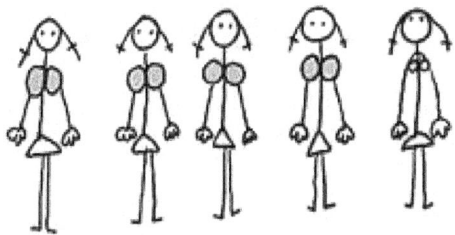

There is another sign to look for, but not to get alarmed about, is sluggish body activity known as "breasts deferred." It could be nothing or in some cases the cause may be related to some hormonal imbalance. This can usually be resolved by, proper examination, along with the right hygienic program. Keeping the body clean during this time is very important. It brings satisfying results and relief from any potential problems.

The size of the mature breasts cannot be predicted during this stage. Another season they must enter to achieve their ultimate destination. As the breasts are waiting for their right time in this stage, it reminds me of how we must wait patiently and keep watching for the signs that summer is not far away.

## *Summer*

## YOUTH/ADOLESCENT STAGE

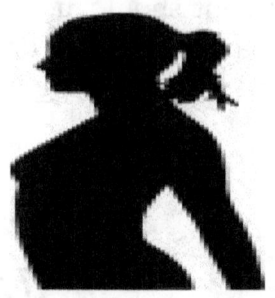

**WHAT'S GOING ON:** Spring has gone and summer opens before us. March winds and April showers have done their work and the seeds we have carefully put into the earth are making their appearance, while others are thirsting for the gentle showers to awaken them to life. All the beautiful in nature seems to be upon a strife to see which can vie with the other in contributing to our pleasure and happiness, by their buds and blossoms of every hue. Everything in nature is diligent, and moving steadily onward, setting us an example.

In this stage, the breasts, too, are making major adjustments and continuous changes. These visible signs are not to be thought of as its time for the cosmetic accessories or props for the female ego. Rather, blossoming time has come and the body is ready to be-decked with the beauty of breasts.

As the breasts begin to swell and blossom out from the chest, there may be some aches and pains. Nevertheless, this is a normal part of breast development. This phase is called puberty – the period in which one of the tangible evidences is breast growth. As a youth, there is an awareness of physical changes to the body, but mentally, it can be considered a critical phase.

Since the physical changes can vary widely, starting as early as 13 years old, but can range from ages 11 to 16, simple explanations in a calm and reassuring manner can soothe those bewildering new sensations and reactions. It can take an entire season or stage, differing from female to female, for the breasts to mature. In most cases, the nipple enlarges, becomes darker in color, and breast tissue forms beneath it. The glands, that secrete milk, bud off from the milk ducts to increase the amount of fat the female has. A Scripture passage that clarifies this thought is found in Ezekiel 16:7: *"I have caused thee to multiply as the bud of the field, ...thy breasts are fashioned..."*

In this stage, simultaneously, other parts of the body are activating changes, like the endocrine system. It manufactures hormones, whose functions are many. Various hormones initiate, maintain and control the changes in female breasts during puberty. Also, they regulate the menstrual cycle and support pregnancy and breastfeeding. During this stage, the breast tissue is highly sensitive to female hormones — chemical agents that are produced by the ovaries and other tissues. In fact, this whole process is intended to remind the young lady about the role she is approaching. And while the body is preparing itself for that role, it promotes a physical and mental awareness on the way to womanhood.

The approach to the subject of breast awareness is necessarily different for the preadolescent girl than during infancy and childhood. The preadolescent has a different incentive for knowledge before her. The incentive is embedded in the young girl's desire to become a beautiful and capable woman.

At a time when the body has so many developmental tasks to perform, and changes in the youth's physical, mental, and spiritual life, it is of the utmost importance to keep nudging them onto a more health conscious path. Proper bathing, adequate sleep, good thoughts, and good nourishing food are some of the vital aids.

Summer brings with it many variables. It is never a short season. With it comes the hot sun, longer days, a desire for cool air, blooming flowers, and growing gardens. As the young woman is entering womanhood, the breasts breathe --- *long time waited for, and now we're here!*

## *Autumn*

## ADULTHOOD STAGE

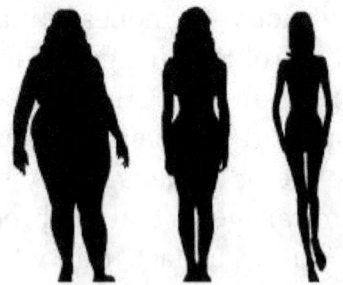

**WHAT'S GOING ON:** The matured breasts have been prepared for this time, waiting on the course they will follow. If that time is pregnancy, the experience is a season of changes.　If not, the breasts remain in a normal state, except during the menstruation period.　　Take note of this Scripture, *"I [am] a wall, and **my breasts like towers**: then was I in his eyes as one that found favour."* (Song of Solomon 8:10).　Yes,  the breasts are standing upright and firm.

If pregnancy has occurred, it creates whole new changes for the breasts.　They awaken out of their rest and may increase three times their normal size.　This acquires the task of enlargement with the skin glands and　the　areolas around  the  nipples grow larger and darker.

The pigmented area around the nipples are tiny glands that take on new growth and appear as little bumps.　Secretion gradually forms.　The appearance of one or more swellings in the armpit or adjacent area is not unusual.　This is due to breast-like tissue situated in abnormal areas undergoing similar changes to those of the breasts.

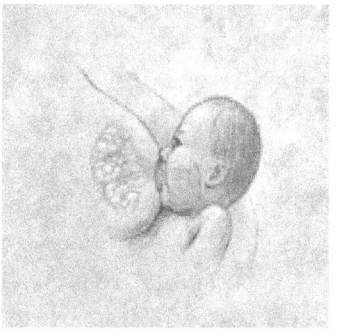

Toward the end of pregnancy and just before childbirth, an abundant secretion of a whitish opaque substance, discharging continuously from the nipples should be noticed by the woman.　That is called colostrums.　The breasts now contain a milk reservoir at childbirth to breastfeed.

Breastfeeding is a natural extension of pregnancy – so the mother's body can nourish the infant.　Isaiah 66:11 sheds light on this, *"That ye may suck, and be satisfied with the breasts of her consolations; that ye may milk out, and be delighted with the abundance of her glory."*　Other Scripture passages amplify this thought, too.　Breastfeeding is the easiest, simplest and most inexpensive way to feed a baby. Also, it offers many health benefits to both mother and infant.　Breast milk is essential to the life and well-being of a newborn.

Although lactation is an automatic physiological proc-ess, breastfeeding is a learned behavior. Little preparation is required and physical obstacles are rare, However, suc-cessful breastfeeding requires adequate nutrition and rest.

Overall, the physical changes speed up as women con-tinue in this stage, but even by middle age, the breasts are still capable of milk production and breastfeeding. How-ever, they may become smaller as shrinkage of the milk glands occur. It differs from woman to woman.

Before entering into the next stage, you may see some drooping of the breasts, but it shouldn't be a cause to alarm. While breasts don't have muscle tissue, they do get sup-port from ligaments. Gravity, weight gain, and excessive bouncing all contribute to the elongating of these ligaments. Consider activities that strengthen your chest and core, to help keep the breasts looking youthful.

It's harvest time, which brings a bounty of fruits and vegetables, along with changing and falling leaves. If you're contemplating breast enhancement surgery, don't rush it. Rather fall in line with what nature has given you.

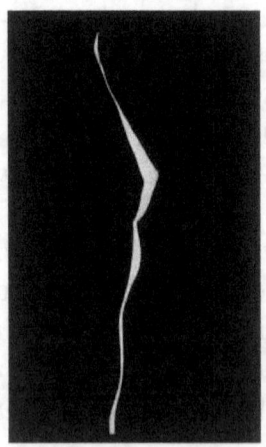 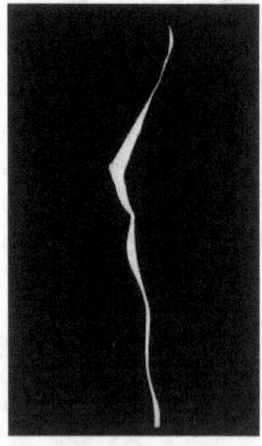

*Winter*

## SENIOR ADULT/ELDERLY STAGE

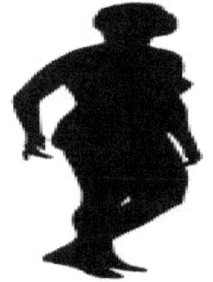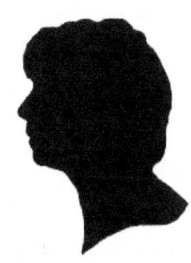

**WHAT'S GOING ON:** Weather that numbs the toes and freezes the nose makes everyone want to stay indoors. Like the winter season, the breasts experience chilling realities, such as sagging, wrinkling skin, and flattening out. Moreover, they may lose some tone and firmness, too. This can be likened unto winter's unwanted "weather like" conditions, that are prone to exist during this stage. It's little wonder why winter gets a bad rap. But the warmth of it all is, women's breasts can still be winterized despite the weatherizing.

Every woman, no matter who she is, will sooner or later experience menopause if her life is extended. It is not a curse; it is a beautiful, wholesome, natural change of life. As the Scripture states, *"The hoary head is a crown of glory, if it be found in the way of righteousness."* Proverbs 16:31. But because the level of health in the world has degenerated to such a low level, menopause instead has been termed a disease. To the contrary, literally speaking, it refers to a woman's last period.

This season's unwelcomed guests come in the door with

its annoying symptoms, just like the menopausal "curses" as some have coined them.   Namely, hot flashes, night sweats, sleep difficulties, vaginal dryness, skin changes, hair loss, mood swings, and weight gain. Menopause does not trigger these symptoms, but an unhealthy lifestyle. As a result, the breasts are affected.   To avoid menopause is like skipping over winter, which cannot happen. Instead, rid the body of these unwelcomed symptoms, and nature can do its work without interruption.

If rightly represented, this stage can be looked upon as the woman's climacteric time of life – after a metamorphosis of physical changes. Hence, natural menopause is experienced only by a few women because of the high rate of hysterectomies, other surgeries, and medications.

With aging, the breasts are affected by the hormonal change activation -- estrogen and progesterone drops, signaling that the milk ducts and lobes can retire.  Moreover, several of the functioning glands are replaced by fibrous tissue and there is a simultaneous loss of fat tissue and a weakening of the connective tissue that binds all the tissues together.   Let's face it!  The breasts need weatherproofing to help you through this season.   All of the modalities needed can be found in chapter 6.

This can be a great time and one of the rewarding stages of life only by keeping in mind this cold fact that some of the things that happen to the breasts are beyond your control.  Like the saying "ole man winter is here to stay" -- since he's staying, women, learn to make the best of this time by cooperating with nature!

Tis the season to wrap up the breasts structurally and functionally.  Get the picture?   The breasts were no afterthought, but a revelation of "the skillful and wonderful workmanship of the Creator," in season and out of season!

# Chapter 2

## Got Breast Disease?

*Symptoms.  Fear.   Hope.*

For starters, I have no personal experience with breast disease, mainly cancer. The women in my family have all escaped it.  This topic would probably be pretty insignificant, if I was not a medical missionary and had not worked with several females with these conditions.  Notwithstanding, I believe that I am hyper-informed about breast cancer and other breast disorders.  I've come to know the extensive details of the history behind breast cancer treatments, mainly from the Word of God and then from nature where the Native Americans applied mud amalgams containing shreds of spider lilies hundreds of years ago,  to oncologists using prescription drugs derived from the elements in spider lilies today.  Depending on the circumstances, I know that soy, in the diet, can be good or bad.  I know that the reign on mammograms is ever-changing and probably coming to an end and enough to write thousands of words.

As a medical missionary, I find myself consulting with numerous women, giving recommendations and providing a health "protocol" on the various aspects of breast  diseases, especially cancer.  This can be construed that I have an expanded knowledge on the topic,  coming from a woman without a (worldly) medical degree.  But this  doesn't entirely explain  my motivation.

Prior to getting into the medical missionary work, if you asked me about breast cancer or other breast disorders, the conversation wouldn't have lasted a full minute.  I couldn't have told you how it originated, the risk factors, or if there are certain foods that could help prevent it or cause it. I didn't even know much about MY breast anatomy and physiology. Yet I feel partially responsible *for* *"the lack of knowledge,"* (Hosea 4:6) amongst God's people and even in the world and was compelled to write this book.

Breasts health should become a common topic. Why? Conditions and the times demand it. The subject of breast disease, especially cancer, can be discussed from any of several points of view. Yet many women approach it with varied and mixed emotions. Few women plan for it and even fewer of them want to discuss it. Breast cancer alone affects a woman's whole life –physically, mentally, and spiritually, along with her family.

The idea of females and breast disease, such as cancer, just does not happen when you turn 50 or wake up one morning. Neither does it happen "just because." An accidental disease -- there's no such thing. As it turns out, breast disease, mainly cancer, is a reality and it is a word feared by many women. The true horror comes in the fact that the majority of women faced with this crisis are unknowledgeable, as to "how" and "what" to do. Many are faced with a task beyond their wisdom and understanding. Yet, it is when a woman comes face to face with this type of situation, she realizes the crisis. Is breast cancer "a disaster waiting to happen?" Here's a horror story of a baby who was a victim of the results of breast cancer:

*(NBC Today Show):* <u>*Toddler Aleisha Hunter Among Youngest to Survive Breast Cancer*</u> *-- " Two years ago, Aleisha Hunter got breast cancer, making her one of the nearly 300,000 new annual cases to surface. The difference? Aleisha was a 2-and-a-half-year-old toddler when the small lump developed in*

*her chest. Doctors diagnosed her with juvenile breast carcinoma when she was only 3. Over time, little Aleisha's tumor became very painful. Her mom, Melanie, says her daughter "wasn't eating, she wasn't sleeping." So doctors performed what is called a <u>radical modified mastectomy</u>, in which they removed the little girl's entire breast and the lymph nodes under her arm. "It's hard to imagine a mastectomy in a 3-year-old," Dr. Egler says. "But these are definitely treated with surgery. In terms of doing a complete mastectomy, I suspect that it comes from the fact that there's so little breast tissue in a 3-year-old that it might have been the default." Still, the child remembers the ordeal, and seems to understand what she went through. "I had breast cancer," she tells "Today" quietly. Her mom says she'll need reconstructive surgery when she gets older."* **Reported by AOL Health on January 20, 2011.**

This heartrending story is full of shocking descriptions that naturally bring out a heap of emotions. On the surface, this is but a sample of the alarming occurrences that happen as a result of breast cancer. I'm very disturbed when I read or hear an account of still another medical horror story. Could this little girl been rescued from this experience? The answer is yes. You will find the anecdotes in this book.

Breast cancer is a headliner disease and it receives more research funding than many other cancers combined. In 1999, the National Cancer Institute spent $126 million more on breast cancer than anything else (AIDS came in second). Not only is breast cancer the most common cancer affecting women, but the numbers steadily climb each year. In our research, we have found that statistically, the number of breast cancer diagnoses among females in their twenties is increasing at a surprising rate. To put it plainly, it shows that a female is never to old — or too young — and the need for help is eminent!

For those who don't know, the United States is said to be one of the wealthiest, most highly educated nations in the world, yet it is one of the sickest. In view of this, data significant to America's breast cancer crisis, among women, is to be noted:

- 1 in 7 will develop breast cancer over course of their lifetimes;
- Each year, more than 200,000 develop the disease and 40,000 succumb to it, making it three times more common than other gynecological cancers
- Breast cancer is the second leading cause of death in women, ages 45-50
- Breast cancer is the number two killer after lung cancer.
- If breast cancer is a part of your family history, your risk is much higher.
- Breast cancer has risen over the past 5 decades.

There you have it ---the shocking truth! Or is it? The true shock comes in the fact that because of the U.S. dominance of marketing, breast disease, particularly cancer has been exported across the world. It was once a disease of the Western world, however, breast cancer has become a global concern. Health communities, country by country, are faced with rising levels of breast cancer cases. Without giving it much thought, the disease has caught up with everyone, especially those countries that have adopted the western civilization lifestyle. In short, it has been labeled the Standard American Way (S.A.W.).

S.A.W. covers a gamut of lifestyle decisions. From what

you eat and drink, how you dress, the environment you live in, all the way to how you are educated. It affects the rich and poor, educated and uneducated, even the young and old. There are no boundaries. When a woman adapts to the S.A.W., she conforms to its activities. These behaviors turn into habits, which develops into a lifestyle. At some point, women must realize how their "lifestyle behaviors," connected to their years of life, play a major role in their health.

Got breast cancer? Sometimes you'll hear people say that breast cancer runs in the family, in other words, it's hereditary. This is one of the causes supported by the medical profession. However, they do not give further details about its hereditary connection.

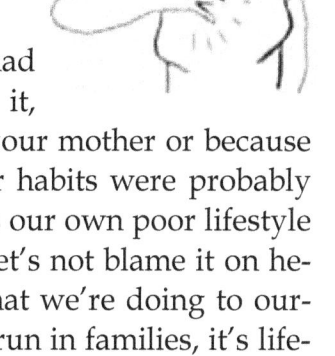

For example, if your mother had breast cancer and then you get it, doesn't mean that you got it from your mother or because of your mother. It means that your habits were probably the same as your mother. In fact, it's our own poor lifestyle choices that bring about disease so let's not blame it on heredity but take responsibility for what we're doing to ourselves. Instead, it isn't disease that run in families, it's lifestyle habits! In chapters 3 and 4, we highlight the S.A.W. lifestyle specifics for your scrutiny.

Before going any further, like women, men can get breast cancer, too. As we have seen, breast cancer is no respecter of person, gender or age. Although this book is mainly female-specific, men can benefit from this information in more ways than one as well.

Despite the overwhelming evidence that the United States approach to breast cancer is SERIOUSLY FLAWED, nevertheless, its customs and habits have more nations adapting to them. In recent years, breast cancer has riddled our society for a lot of reasons. In reviewing the history of it, one cannot be impressed with the results. Even with years of research, doctors still know relatively little about the cause of breast cancer or even the other breast disorders. In the concealed female organ—the breasts, minor and even serious conditions can exist without causing pain, bleeding or other symptoms. Many of the breast diseases are presented in different ways. Each exhibits different symptoms.

In order to better understand the identity of breast cancer and other breast disorders, I use "medical" data to lay out the details. In doing this, I am not saying that I agree with everything it says but to allow everyone to *"judge for yourselves."*

Breast cancer is classified into two **types**, and they are noninvasive (DCIS) and invasive. **(DCIS means ductal carcinoma in situ.)** In addition, breast cancer has been further classified according to what type of tissue it arises from i.e., milk ducts, connective tissues, milk producing lobules.

The medical society has put breast cancer into four stages. Generally, a higher stage tends to mean a worse prognosis in the eyes of the doctor. Contrarily, no matter what stage your breast cancer is at the time of diagnosis, it does not tie the Great Physician's hands. Remember, *"it is the Lord that healeth you."* (Exodus 15:26).

## OTHER BREAST DISORDERS

Although the majority of the disorders of the female breast are benign in character, the breast is one of the two female organs that are most frequently the primary site of cancer. The breast normally changes during menstruation, pregnancy, lactation, and menopause.

Names given for other breast disorders are as follows:
- Fat Necrosis
- Fibroadenoma
- Fibrocystic
- Mastitis

**Additionally you can** find a short description about each one in the Glossary.

Basically, breast cancer and other breast disorders is a process that follows a course of actions. In order to avoid this course, one must be the pilot of that ship. For instance, as a pilot, you would chart a safe course and heed danger signals. So it is with breast diseases. You should both know the signals and heed the warnings. Then, the basic question to introduce such discussion seems to be "What are the signals and warnings?

The signs of breast disease are those changes that can be observed objectively by the individual. Considering these changes, in combination with other symptoms, can speak breast cancer and other breast disorders. Some signs or symptoms can be

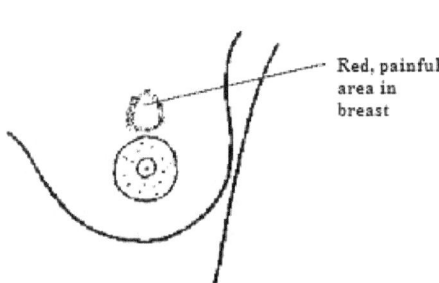

Red, painful area in breast

confused with other conditions.  Many lives have been kept

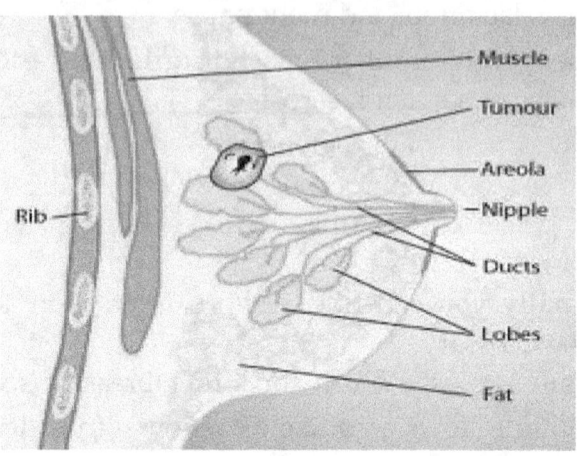

safe by recognizing warning signals of possible breast disease (cancer) and taking proper action.  In fact, many more lives can be saved by knowing the warning signs.

For your own protection, it is imperative to know the danger signals.  Remember, however, that these signals do

**ILLUSTRATION OF SYMPTOMS OF BREAST CANCER**

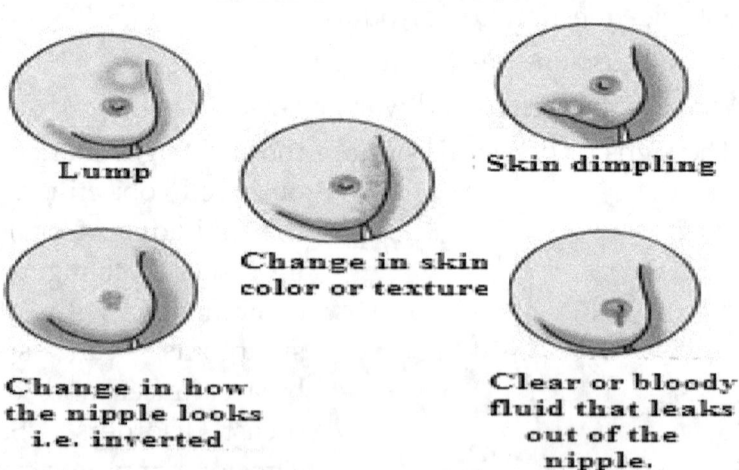

not always indicate cancer. Rather, they may be only signs that something is wrong — and some type of action is required. On the other hand, sometimes fear may cause a person to experience symptoms associated with their breasts. Overall, all signals or symptoms demand attention.

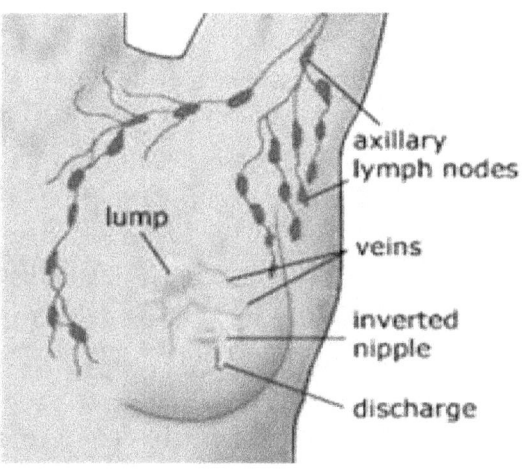

Warning signals of breast cancer and other breast disorders include, but are not limited to:

- Swollen lymph nodes or lumps on the underarm,
- Red, sore, tender, tingling, or swollen breast
- Nipple changes or discharge
- Pain in the back
- Differences in size, shape, or color
- Ulcers, Infection, Inflammation
- Bumps, lumps, dimples in breasts
- Itchy, burning, scaly, crusty skin on nipple

These are nature's red lights, some of the danger signals. An alarming aspect is that sometimes these symptoms will leave on its own. This occurs only, if nature is al-

lowed to take its course, without interruption or hin-
drance, to correct serious defects in your life. The symptoms can be corrected by allowing nature to do its
work. If not, an attack on the breasts is in progress and it
can be with a vengeance.

The more you know about the warning signs of breast
cancer and breast disorders, the better prepared you will be
to act quickly. Moreover, both are created equally, by lifestyle habits, and can be deadly.

On the whole, breast cancer is weak compared to God.
There is no need to fear or worry, for the Bible tells us that:
*"For to him that is joined to all the living, there is hope; for a liv-
ing dog is better than a dead lion."* Ecclesiastes 9:4. In other
words, where there is life there is hope. May the following
lines encourage and strengthen you:

> **"To all who are reaching out to feel "To all who
> are reaching out to feel the guiding hand of God,
> the moment of greatest discouragement is the
> time when divine help is nearest."** *Desire of Ages,
> p. 528.*

# Chapter 3

## *A Cause For Concern*

*Physically.   Mentally.   Spiritually.*

As breast cancer grows rampant in society today, there are many reasons for the epidemic. Studies after studies have given us clues about the factors contributing to this lurking disease. An unveiling of these factors will help unlock the mysteries that still linger today and help sum up the causes.

The Scripture declares *"...and the <u>cause</u> which I knew not I searched out."* (Job 29:16). Searching for the cause of all breast diseases require the known and unknown. It involves a strict, close, diligent, deep-rooted search, as digging for gold. When you find any treasure, have it in your possession, you take ownership of it. Likewise with breast cancer and other breast disorders, you cannot rest content with having a superficial understanding about it but you need to be in control of it.

As we trace from cause to effect, you may or may not be aware of the challenges of breast cancer, but at the same time, many are  seriously unaware of how their choices in lifestyle are connected to them, and how these choices are the major contributing factors, to a large degree, for sickness and disease.

Considering the cause, we must insert here Proverbs 26:2, *"As the bird by wandering, as the swallow by flying, so the curse causeless shall not come."*   In other words, *"we reap what we sow"* (Galatians 6:7-8). This Scripture is known as the law of the harvest. Oftentimes, we are recipients of what we have done or others have done i.e., parents, ancestors, and the effect of what was done may be a part of the experience. There are some key factors that contribute to the harvest that have been planted which manifests itself in the female breasts. In this section we highlight some of these factors, however, breast cancer and other breast disorders are not limited to these only. The desire is to feature those "lifestyle" choices that are practiced in our day-to-day living. They are diet, emotional, spiritual and environmental factors. Not all encompassing, it can take one, two, or all factors to breakdown the body, resulting in breast disease.

## DIET FACTOR

Diet has become a four letter word with a S.A.D. history. S.A.D. means Standard American Diet and it has been and is a controlling factor in many lives. To some, it's just a word describing a part of their lifestyle. A look at Webster 1828 dictionary defines DIET, *n.* 1. Food or victuals; DIET, *v.* 1. To eat; to feed.

Most of the world would say that America is one of the best fed nations on earth. Best fed is relative, especially. if based on the average American's diet. In the assembling of facts to undergird this issue, a study revealed the essence of the average American diet. They,

- Consume 300 soft drinks a year, and each of those soft drinks has about 12 teaspoons of sugar.
- Consume over 170 pounds of sugar a year, including 400 candy bars, 500 donuts, numerous cookies, pastries, and cakes.
- Will eat over 12 entire 3,000 pound cows in their lifetime.
- Eat 6 entire pigs, 3,000 chickens and other birds, 3,000 assorted fish and sea creatures, and drink over

30,000 quarts of milk in their lifetime.

- Have a sodium (salt) intake of 4,000 mg/day (250 mg/day minimum necessary level & 2,400 mg/day maximum with normal blood pressure)
- Use unsaturated, polyunsaturated hydrogenated and/or partially hydrogenated oils, such as margarine, lard, shortening, butter, vegetable, canola, etc.

The average American, moreover women, are included in this data. As you digest all of this "food-wise" information, keep in mind the S.A.D. history.

People are eating more and more refined, processed, and packaged foods. Most packaged foods are fortified with vitamins and minerals but our bodies cannot assimilate these added-on vitamins. Most package foods contain 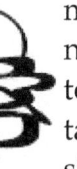 more sugar, salt, and fat than we need. Many are full of chemicals to keep the food looking and tasting fresh. Food is a necessity; however, it has become a 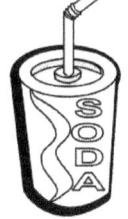 master, -- yes a tyrant! Hence, nutritious food feeds us in every way – not only physically, but mentally and spiritually. The problem comes when food becomes an obsession, it can become the death of people, as stated in this quote:

**"Only when we are intelligent in regard to the principles of healthful living, can we be fully aroused to see the evils resulting from improper diet."** *Counsels on Diet and Foods, p.24.*

Beliefs about food can be hard to change. But here's "food for thought" for you to chew on – **Health is a gold mine; Not a nugget!**

## EMOTIONAL FACTORS

Today, Americans are leading more stressful lives, brought on by war, the sluggish economy, natural disasters, and juggling work and family issues. And when their stress level rises, a growing number of them become sick. As they seek relief from stress, more Americans are swallowing a pill or drinking alcohol. Stress is not the situation itself—but our response to it. Hence, STRESS has a human face.

To some, brain chemistry is a complicated subject; however, some facts are clear with regard to the physiology of the brain. First, there is an intimate relationship between body function and the mind. The mind is known to be able to affect in any way, any type of activity that the body is capable of performing. Proverbs 4:23 speaks to this, *"Keep thy heart with all diligence; for out of it [are] the issues of life."* Different emotional reactions can affect an involuntary type of body function. Anger can cause an increase in blood pressure; fright, a rapid pulse; and extreme nervousness,

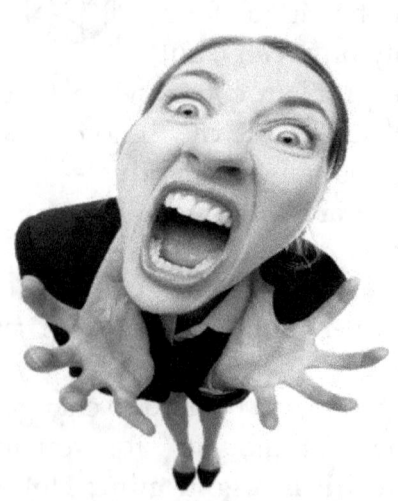

biting of fingernails. Naturally, there are also other physiologic changes with each of these states. Therefore, it is evident that there is a definite and important interconnection among the organs of the body and an interaction that is intimate and all encompassing.

This union of bodily of responses is affected by the dominance of the central nervous system that controls, in addition to all the nerves of the body, the glands of internal secretion, the action of the blood vessels, and the function of the vital organs — heart, liver and kidneys. Fear knows little bounds in its effect on the body. The tongue can refuse to speak and the legs can become powerless. Even more significant is the role that fear can play in breast disease, mainly cancer. The frightened female develops a state of fear that in some way raises the threshold of the disease, thereby heightening the condition and pain.

Other familiar words that are negative exposures include bitterness, cruelty, doubt, envy, guilt, hatred, ill-will, jeal-

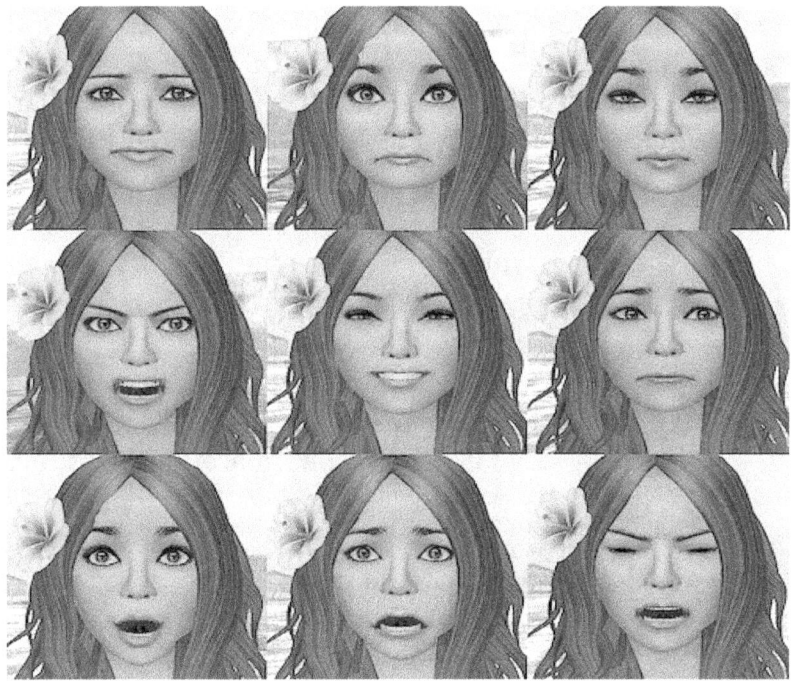

ousy, lust, anxiety, malice, over-sensitive, depression, panic, quarrelsome, resentment, stress, tension, unforgiving, vindictiveness, and worry. Some of these may appear to be out of your control, but many clearly are not. They cause the body to produce toxic material, via the hormones, which weakens the immune system and allows cancer to form in the body. In women, the breasts are one of the areas it manifests itself in.

Unmistakably, emotional factors not only bring on disease, they can cause death. They are physical, mental, and spiritual destroyers!

## ENVIRONMENTAL FACTORS

Some female diseases can be caused by the introduction of chemicals to the body. They come in many sources that breakdown the immune system. Just about everything we use, touch, or that's around us can be the culprit. Many expose themselves to chemicals sometimes knowingly and unknowingly. It really can be a situation of an "unseen" sign of "beware," "danger zone," or "enter at your own risk."

The use of chemical agents is becoming a way of life in our nation, and even across the world. Chemicals, or to use another familiar word, preservatives are used in cosmetics, clothing, food and pharmaceutical products, disrupt the body functions. Other culprits include aspirin and other painkillers, over the counter prescription drugs, tobacco, alcohol, commercially grown vegetables that contain pesticide and commercially raised cattle and poultry, because they are fed with estrogen – like chemicals.

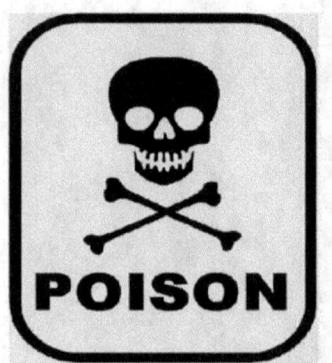

But one of the most significant features is synthetic hormone replacement therapy (HRT). According to a study published online in the Journal of the National Cancer Institute, **breast cancer rates for women dropped in tandem with decreased use of HRT**. This supports existing evidence that HRT is linked with breast cancer, which is an estrogen-related cancer. So it is no surprise that giving women potent synthetic estrogens will increase their risk.

There are similar risks for younger women who use oral contraceptives — birth control pills, which are also comprised synthetic hormones — have been linked to **cervical and breast cancers**.

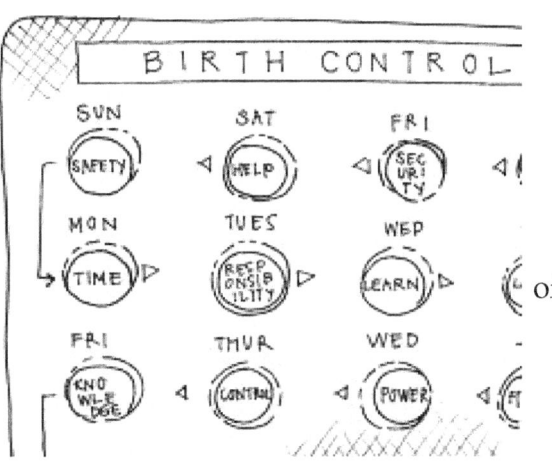

Another aggravating aspect in breast cancer is, unfortunately, the breast cancer screening tool itself, namely mammograms, which is discussed in chapter 6.

Overall, poisonous substances, such as chemicals, when introduced into the body, cause great damage in a variety of ways. They put the body on emergency status. These chemicals have a very definite, and for some, very dangerous effect. In women, what it boils down to is that these chemicals affect your hormone systems and can cause a whole array of effects

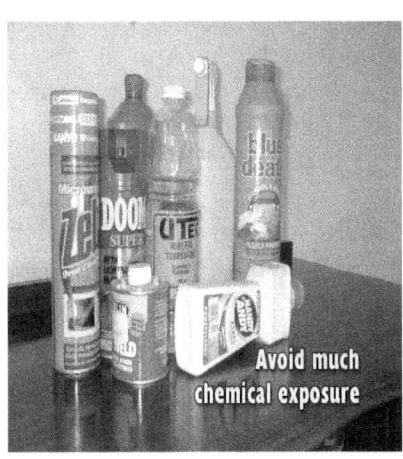

Avoid much chemical exposure

in your breasts. As busy women, we seek conveniences and industries are very adept at finding substances that make life easier for us.

By no means are these all of the factors that cause disease in females. These barely scraped the surface. There are more questionable factors to be on the lookout for. We have some homework to do as stated in Ecclesiastes 1:13: *"And I gave my heart to seek and search out by wisdom concerning all [things] that are done under heaven: this sore travail hath God given to the sons of man to be exercised therewith."* Hence, what you have been informed about thus far, consider it a start for you to investigate and see if any of these factors are featured in your lifestyle.

## SPIRITUAL FACTORS

Lord, why are Christians sick? At one time, this had been my question. I even pondered the thought, if Christians have the same diseases and sicknesses as non-Christians, why serve God? Unsurprisingly, I found the answer why God allows people to get sick — Christians and non-Christians — based on following three reasons;

- **For the glory of God:** *John 9:1-3 – "And as Jesus passed by, He saw a man which was blind from birth. And the disciples asked Him saying, Master, who did sin, this man or his parents, that he was born blind? And Jesus answered, Neither hath this man sinned, nor his parents, but that the works of God should be made manifest in him."* **What then should a person do?** *"Not that I speak in respect of want: for I have learned, in whatsoever state I am, [therewith] to be content."* (Philippians 4:11). Therefore, all the praying in the world will not remove an affliction for the glory of God, unless God wills it.

44

- **Because of unconfessed sins:** *1 Corinthians 11:28 - "But let a man examine himself, and so let him eat of [that] bread, and drink of [that] cup. For he that eateth and drinketh unworthily, eateth and drinketh damnation to himself, not discerning the Lord's body. For this cause many [are] weak and sickly among you, and many sleep.* **What then should a person do?** *"If we confess our sins, he is faithful and just to forgive us [our] sins, and to cleanse us from all unrighteousness."* (1 John 1:9). *"For if we would judge ourselves, we should not be judged. But when we are judged, we are chastened of the Lord, that we should not be condemned with the world."* (1 Corinthians 11:31-32). Sickness because of sin is a judgment by God, but it can be removed if we make things right with Him. All the praying in the world will not heal the affliction caused by sin, unless it is the prayer of repentance by the believer who has sinned.

- **Violations of God's natural laws:** *1 Corinthians 3:16-17 – "Know ye not that ye are the temple of God, and [that] the Spirit of God dwelleth in you? If any man defile the temple of God, him shall God destroy; for the temple of God is holy, which [temple] ye are."* *1 Corinthians 6:19-20 – "What? know ye not that your body is the temple of the Holy Ghost [which is] in you, which ye have of God, and ye are not your own? For ye are bought with a price: therefore glorify God in your body, and in your spirit, which are God's."*

What then should a person do? **"The strange absence of principle which characterizes this generation, and which is shown in their disregard of the laws of life and health, is astonishing. Ignorance prevails upon this subject, while light is shining all around them. With the majority, their principal anxiety is, What shall I eat? what shall I drink? and wherewithal shall I be clothed? Notwithstanding all that is said and written in regard to how we should treat our bodies, appetite is the great law which governs men and women generally."** *3 Testimonies,*

**p. 140.**

There is a view held by some that spirituality is a detriment to health. This is the sophistry of Satan. The religion of the Bible is not detrimental to the health of either body or mind. The influence of the Spirit of God is the very best medicine for disease as stated in 3 John 2, *it says "Beloved, I wish above all things that thy prosper and be in health, even as thy soul prospereth."*

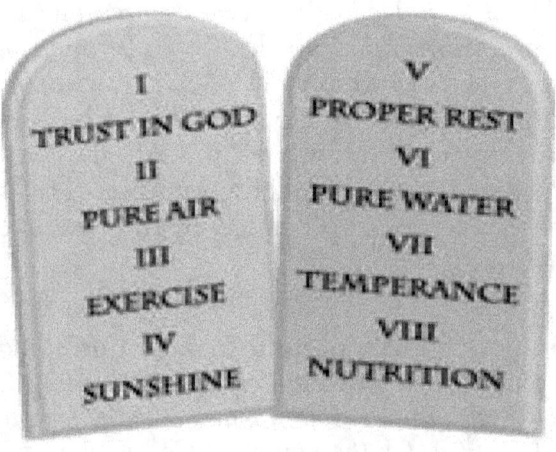

This church and the world is out of joint. It needs today what it needed over two thousand years ago--a revelation of Christ. A great work of reform is demanded, and it is only through the grace of Christ that the work of restoration, physical, mental, and spiritual, can be accomplished. Sickness, suffering, and death are work of an antagonistic power. Satan is the destroyer; God is the restorer.

# Chapter 4

## The Big Cover-up

*Protection. Confinement. Comfort.*

So far, we have covered some vital things – but there is a lot yet to come! As we keep digging away, it will be tempting to ignore some of the information in previous sections as we move forward – don't let it happen. Knowledge is progressive. Every step builds on the ones before, and it is only as you continue that you can move on and be enlightened on many more pertinent things.

When it comes to breast diseases, largely cancer, some may think every woman is at risk. That is absolutely false. The truth is that every woman can succumb to the risk factors and end up with breast cancer and/or the other breast disorders. Although the risk of getting breast cancer continues to climb every year, a certain percentage of women are determined not to be a victim — directly or indirectly.

In this section, it's time to uncover an area of a woman's life that few consider a problem. That is DRESS: thefemale's secret weapon! Aiming at the breasts, we will expose the under and outer garments, beauty and hygienic products, and show how women daily pull the trigger on their health – some knowingly, others unknowingly.

Millions of dollars are spent each year in America, even now in other parts of the world, urging women to buy this or that clothing, or insisting on the need for certain cosmetics. When it comes to clothing or cosmetics, namely, fashion, everyone's got an opinion. While many focus on these fashions, few understand, or even think about the health implications. Years back, when someone was dressed fashionably, a compliment was made to that person saying, "You are dressed to kill!" Surprisingly, little did the person know that statement was aligned with truth!

For all humans, dress should be treated as a necessity of life. This has logic. Nature teaches us that it is God who provides for us, and that, as we come to Him, He can give us that which we need in order to live. In relation to dress, a verse of Scripture comes to mind. Genesis 3:21: *"Unto Adam also and to his wife did the LORD God make coats of skins, and clothed them."*

**"The atmosphere was changed. It was no longer unvarying as before the transgression. God clothed them with coats of skins to protect them from the sense of chilliness and then of heat to which they were exposed."** *Story of Redemption, p. 46.*

After sin, the Creator provided a garment for the two. Initially humans are born nude, however, our dress today is derived from choosing a wardrobe of our parents or own liking, diversified with color coded preferences.

Women who wish to pay proper regard to their health must give attention to their dress. Not only the clothing they put on, but the various toiletries and cosmetics used for feminine hygiene and to enhance beauty. Why? Whenever these are allowed to diminish in even one manner from the beauty and utility of health, it creates problems.

Healthy dress permits every organ in the body to perform its functions undisturbed. No garment worn should ever be allowed to interfere with entire freedom of movement, or with the natural action of any bodily organ, or with the perfectly free circulation of the blood. The general rule of dress is to have all garments as loose in fashion as is consistent with bodily comfort, and allow the most perfect freedom in the exercise of every muscle of the body. On the other hand, dress should be used to moderate the extremes of heat or cold, according to the climate of the wearer and the weather. Clothing, therefore, which the usages of society, and the severity of climates render indispensable, should as an invariable rule, is loose as possible without bodily discomfort. Women must learn to see the danger, if not the hideousness of going against this principle.

A statement by a favorite author, Ellen G. White set forth a concept regarding women diseases.

**"Half of the diseases of women are caused by unhealthful dress."** *Healthful Living, page 123.*

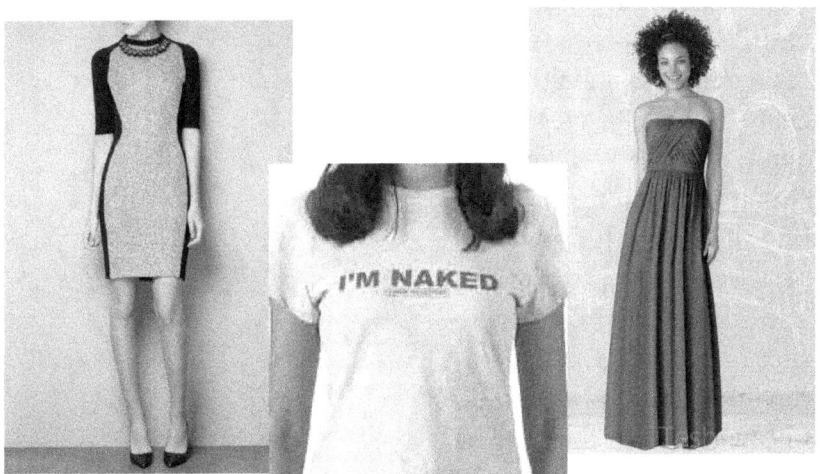

Health should be the paramount law of dress; comfort should always coincide with health. To the eye of an intelligent observer, nothing should ever be looked upon as beautiful, that proves to be offensive and interferes with either. By a contrary arrangement, women still choose to dress fashionably, no matter how dangerous it may prove. More consequences are now attached to figure and form than to health and comfort.

On the other hand, some women are on the right tract regarding their dress, but there is still a lot to be learned. Armed with the necessary tools, they would be better prepared on what to look for and wear. More significantly, the core of the matter covers the deeper paths of dress. It may take a while for some to sit down and say, "out of sight"; "out of mind" does matter, especially when what's underneath can make all the difference.

Let's start with something familiar to women -- the brassiere, also known as the "bra." It is an undergarment worn to cover women's breasts. Its origin can be traced back to the early 1900's. However during that time, a more prevalent undergarment was being worn--the corset. As a result of health concerns and warnings against the wearing of corsets, warnings posed by tight clothing, were beneficial in putting an end to the corset, or were they? Many women today might be shocked to know, they could be wearing the corset's descendant every day, in the form of the modern bra.

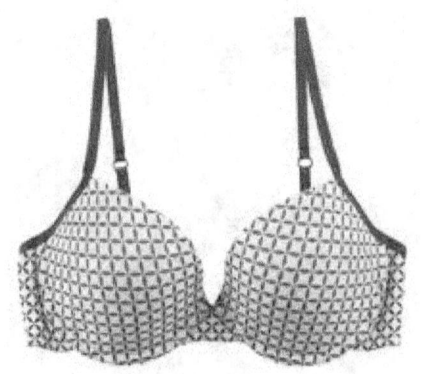

The metal under-wire of a bra and the clasps and straps that keep it in place evolved directly from the stays and clasps of corsets. What links them both together is — they are seen as an essential undergarment, and the same kind of support is offered. It's a thought to ponder.

Since the bra's inception, its revolving evolution has

made its way into society, in the name of fashion. There are several different types of bras worn for different purposes.

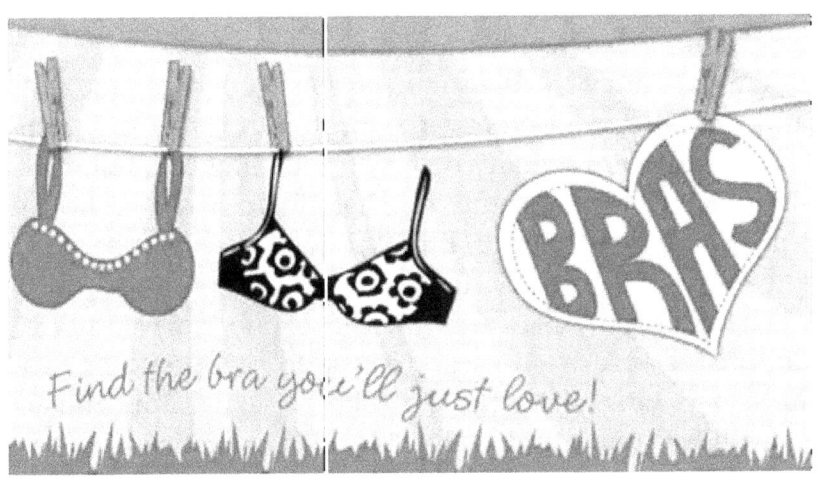

*Find the bra you'll just love!*

You have the "training," "sports," "push up", "underwire", "strapless", "long line, " and "18 hours" just to name a few. Hold tight! In the name of fashion, a certain amount of suffering is borne by women when they wear the bra. It may be gentle to the breasts, but hazardous to your health. The hazards are but not limited to, hindering the circulation of blood and drainage of the lymphatic vessels; worn tightly, it inhibits normal breathing; its tension causes modification of the body; and it locks away the breasts, in a laced-up confinement.

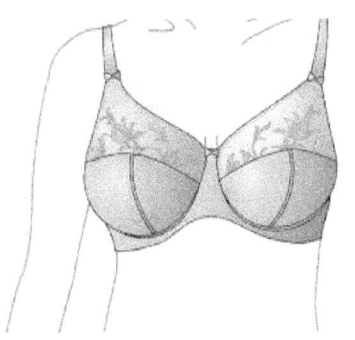

It is an obvious physiological fact, that the chest should have free room to expand itself, and allow the lungs to fill with air. The breathing should meet no resistance from what is worn on the body. The circulation of the blood in the breasts must be perfectly free from any constraint, and for these reasons any garments that press down on the breasts are harmful. Therefore, the physical consequences of these hazards affect the health immeasurably.

Unknowingly by many, the breasts were made to "self-support." Before fashion authenticated the wearing of the bra, women were actually better off retaining the similitude with which the Creator molded them in, rather than the destruction of beauty and life through its ever changing styles.

The main purpose in the design of the bra was not to support the breasts. Instead, it was to accentuate or provide a reducing effect for the sake of sexual appearance. Many full figured and heavy breasted women might say that to go "bra-less" could be painful, uncomfortable, and unacceptable. Yes, some physical discomfort may be experienced. However, we must recall that comfort is very much a matter of habit, and does not make a proper discrimination between the natural sensation of health and the morbid sensitiveness produced by false customs.

On the other hand, small breasted women often use bras that are padded in various ways to make the bust seem larger or more elevated. Padded or contour (lightly padded or lined) bras lead to congestion of the breasts and a higher incidence of disease. (They also bear "false witness.") You will do well to recognize the value of the counsel that advises,

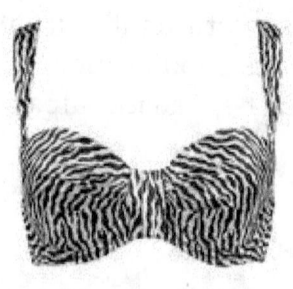

**"Because it is the fashion, many females place**

over their breasts paddings (bras), to give the form the appearance of well-developed breasts. These appendages attract the blood to the chest, and produce a dry, irritating heat. The veins, because of unnatural heat, become contracted, and the natural circulation is obstructed. These appendages, in connection with other bad habits of dressing and eating, result in obstructing the process of nature, making a healthy development of the breasts impossible. And if these become mothers, there cannot be a natural secretion of the fluids, to have a sufficient supply of nourishment for their offspring." *Health Reformer, September 1, 1871.*

The point in all of this is that at the expense of covering up their breasts, too many women are sacrificing their health. It boils down to, without evidence of the reassuring qualities of the bra; women still are persuaded to take unhealthful cover continuously. Unfortunately, custom and habit have a great influence in the lives of many today.

As a custom, and for some time, women have worn the bra for comfort and protection. At night, the bra goes to bed with most women, and the breasts are secure. So you think. Instead, sleeping with a bra is a very risky habit. Not only are the breasts constricted, but the circulation of blood and lymphatics is lessened.

Another risky practice is the selection of an incorrect "cup size," which squeezes the breast tissue and hinders lymphatic drainage. For a quick measurement, slide two fingers under the shoulder straps and the side panels. If the bra is the right size, the fingers should easily slide under it. Wrinkles in the bra, signifies the wrong size. An indicator to use, in the event of discomfort when wearing the bra, is how you feel hours afterward. When the breasts are at their largest and are most tender, the selection of differ-

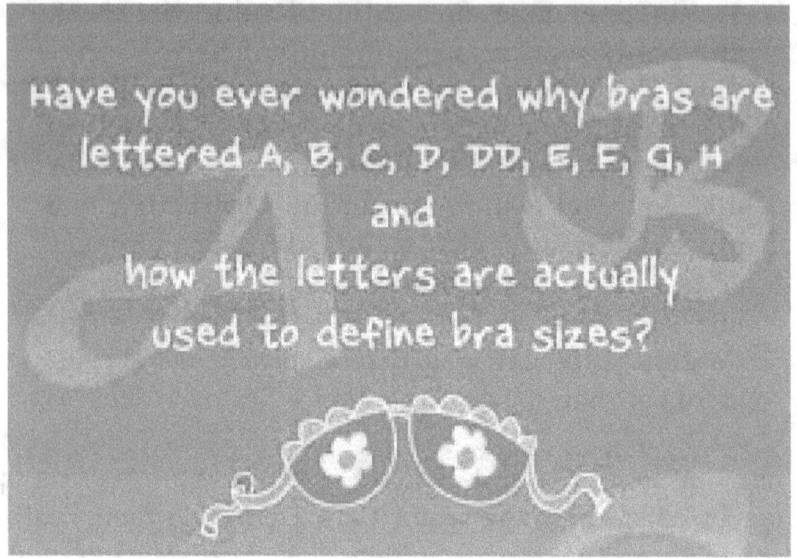

Have you ever wondered why bras are lettered A, B, C, D, DD, E, F, G, H and how the letters are actually used to define bra sizes?

ent bras offers relief, during those special times of the month. To keep in tuned with the breasts much needed relief, maybe you can find peace in the following:

- Do not sleep with the bra on. "Give the breast a rest!"
- Select a bra agreeing with the right cup size, to avoid the "cup running over."

If the bra leaves red marks or grooves on your skin,

- It's too tight and should be "let loose."
- During menstrual cycle, wear a different size bra to accommodate the "changing times."

To sum it up, although a woman uses a thing and likes it, even though she may have used it for years without any apparent injury to herself, that is no proof that it is not an injury to her. A trend, that if we are not careful, this thought can be carried to other lengths which can prove detrimental to the health.

Taking a look at another part of the woman's secret weapon, the view is on what's worn on top or the outer-garment -- mainly the type of fabric. Its makeup is either natural or synthetic fibers. A quick anatomy and physiol-ogy lesson on the skin is worthwhile, since most of the things we wear touch the skin. The skin is the largest organ of the body. It must be allowed to breathe in and out, in order to take in nutrients and release toxins. What is applied to the skin enters the blood stream. It is an

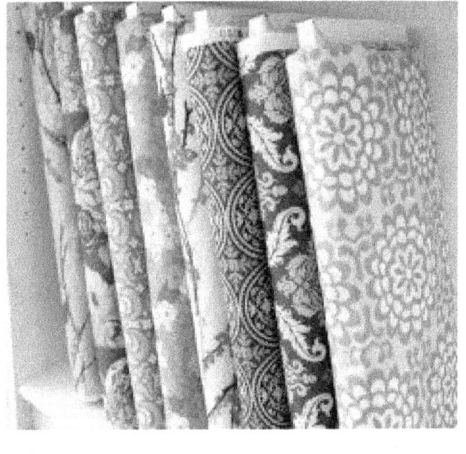

important entryway for substances to the body. While your skin is one of the essential channels for the elimination of toxins, when your skin comes into contact with undesirable substances, they can be absorbed.

Back to natural versus synthetic. They are opposites and possess significant disparity. The many evidences of natu-ral fibers, such as cotton, linen, silk, wool, reveal they should be worn to allow the skin to breathe properly. On the other hand, synthetic fibers, such as polyester, rayon, nylon, acrylic, plastic, reveal they do not allow the pores of the skin to breathe properly, contributing to toxins remain-ing in the breast tissue. Synthetic is anything that is artifi-cial; man-made. A side note -- perhaps the most notorious chemical in today's clothing is formaldehyde.

Formaldehyde is a common ingredient in permanent press formulations, mainly ready-to-wear, no-ironing garments. The out pouring of additives from fabric also means that you inhale air borne toxic substances and take them in through your lungs. These, synthetic fibers and chemicals, create a heavier toxic burden for your body. The short of it, who would think that wearing the wrong fabric exposes the breasts a little bit more
to harmful elements, and are certainly steps toward unhealthy breasts.

After reading about the under and outer-garments, brace yourself for some eye-opening discoveries in personal care products and cosmetics that will make you cringe. You will discover that looking or smelling good could cost not only your breasts, but your body a great deal of misfortune.

**"Many are injuring their <u>health</u> and endangering their lives by using cosmetics…when they become heated…poison is absorbed by the pores of the skin and is thrown in the blood. Many lives have been sacrificed by this means alone."** *Healthful Living, p. 189.2*

A close look at beauty and health products that many put on their skin includes:

| | |
|---|---|
| * Soap | * Powder |
| * Hair Gel | * Lotion |
| * Hair Oil/Grease | * Essential Oils |
| * Body Spray | * Shampoo/Conditioner |
| * Deodorant | * Laundry Detergent |
| * Perfume | * Body Wash |

* Make-up           * Lip Stick/Gloss
* Fingernail Polish    * Hair Dye/Rinse
* Shaving Cream     * Toothpaste
* Perms              * Hair Spray

In no way has this list been exhausted. The enticing advertisements and the bright packages lead many to think they're getting something – which they are really not getting. These marketing pitches seem to promise so much in regards to beauty, hygiene and health. Here, we must be able to read between the lines of the most common claims. Unknowingly, the same products that look so good on the package, they will take over your body – your breasts. Some of the ingredients are POISON!

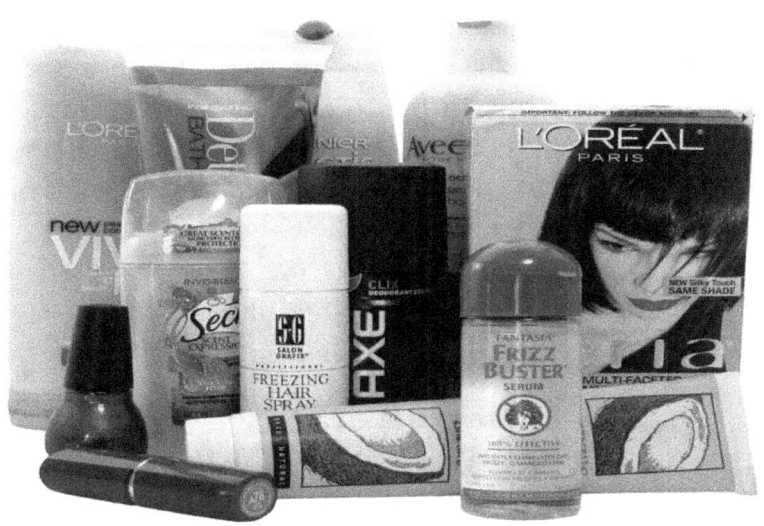

To make an intelligent, healthy selection in cosmetics, it's good to know about the ingredients; because of course... the package probably would never tell you it's poisonous. It's sad there aren't "truth in labeling" laws to clarify some of our cosmetic choices. Understandably, most people would never buy certain products if they knew it contained poison. In other words, if what was really "inside" could actually end up costing you --your life!

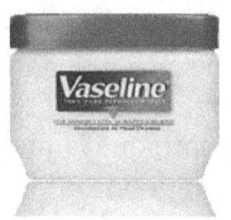
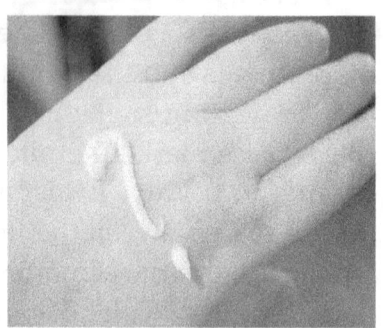

For everything we buy, the ingredients are usually there. Ingredients in skin care and beauty products are listed by the chemical names. For most, the names of these ingredients can be challenging to figure out what they all mean. What's key to know is that the intricate ingredient names are used to cover up the matter, so that none is aware of what one is really buying, unless they obtain a dictionary to find out the meaning of these ingredients. To help you identify them, like an x-ray machine, we will reveal the "inside" of the products' most offending ingredients:

| | |
|---|---|
| * Petroleum Jelly | * Fragrances |
| * Parabens | * Urea |
| * Mineral Oil | * Sodium Lauryl Sulfate |
| * FD&C Color | * Alcohol |
| * Propylene Glycol | * Phthalates |
| * Mineral Oil | * Dimethicone |

These ingredients have been known to cause liver abnormalities, kidney damage, skin irritation, hormonal dysfunctions, birth defects, infertility, cancer, and the lists goes on. What it boils down to is that these "unwanted chemicals" can cause a whole array of effects to the body.

If you find this information to be true, after doing your own research, here are some suggestions to help you transition your personal care products:

- Take an inventory of the cosmetics and toiletries currently in your cupboard.
- Discard of the products whose language has to be decoded.
- Strive to replace those products with "natural" ingredients – healthy replacements.

A word of caution: Beware and take note of the "*safe-for-your healthcare and beauty movement*" that has taken the cosmetics aisle by storm. Everything that is natural is not natural. You must learn the lingo: "natural" versus "organic." Organic is anything that isn't synthetic or man-made. Natural is produced by nature and is indigenous. Bottom line – anything said to be organic or natural is 100%, not 99 ½. On the shelves, natural products are more deceptive to identify. In your decisions of which product is best, your biggest challenge will be narrowing down the flood of choices. An all-natural product should stand out from the rest because it should contain more easily recognizable ingredients, which are few versus many.

Some natural solutions that don't cover up the skin, but treat it naturally include shea butter, olive oil, castor oil, cornstarch, essential oils, castile soap – just to name a few. Surprisingly, most can be found in your kitchen cupboard. We encourage you to keep yourself informed for the sake of your health.

Unfortunately, in this world, many things we enjoy or choose to use can come with potential health risks. Could the "big cover-up" we have shared in this section be looked upon as a conspiracy!  Maybe that's stretching it a bit -- but the best way to avoid any type of deception, use this Scripture as a guide:  *"Finally, brethren, whatsoever things are **true**, whatsoever things [are] **honest**, whatsoever things [are] **just**, whatsoever things [are] **pure**, whatsoever things [are] **lovely**, whatsoever things [are] of **good report**; if [there be] any **virtue**, and if [there be] any **praise**, think on these things."* (Philippians 4:8).

Moreover, a more sure way to "uncover" the unknown is to *"Prove all things, and hold fast to that which is good."* (1 Thessalonians 5:21).

# Chapter 5

## Remove The Cause....Not The Breasts

*Procedure. Impact. Reason.*

These days, risks are taken. Among women, greater risks are taken, in relation to their breasts. In this section, the breast(s) removal syndrome is the focus. Because many women feel they have "zero hope" to be delivered from breast cancer, they result to breast removal. When this surgical procedure is done, it is known to compound female's lives with the pain of "yesterday," mixed with the disappointments and frustrations of "today." It impacts women and their family life dramatically. It means a part of them,

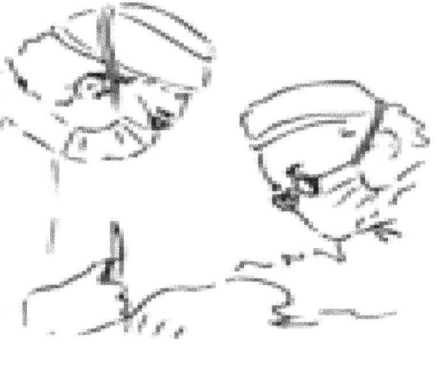

which can never be replaced. But to this matter there is a brighter side that outshines the dark side. Even after a diagnosis has been made or a medical procedure has been performed, there is still much that can be done to regain your health.

On the other hand, breast removal is always more difficult to tolerate when there is no foreseeable future deliverance for doing so. The possibility of lifelong injury or death is not looked upon as too great a risk when opting for this surgical procedure. This treatment of the disease is a nightmare of pain, disfigurement and uncertainty too terrifying to contemplate. It leads most women to accept unpleasant

61

and uncomfortable experiences in anticipation of future hope. Dying for a cure, many breast cancer patients often fall prey to risky results, even at the expense of losing their lives. At the same time it is imperative never to abandon hope!

But how do you distinguish the "hype" from the "hope." Half of the battle is in being informed intellectually. Unless you've done your own research, you should apply caution before using or reacting to any information or another's experience. In essence, when it comes to dealing with "disease" every experience is different. With understanding, information and knowledge leads to protective and lifesaving options. It may be hard, but not impossible, to have a vibrant perspective on this matter.

Although there is a tendency among women to view breast(s) removal as a necessary act of breast cancer, there is no truth to this. In addition, there is no possible advantage in enduring any pain or suffering that can be prevented; instead much harm may result from such a procedure. Unquestionably, there are some serious complica-

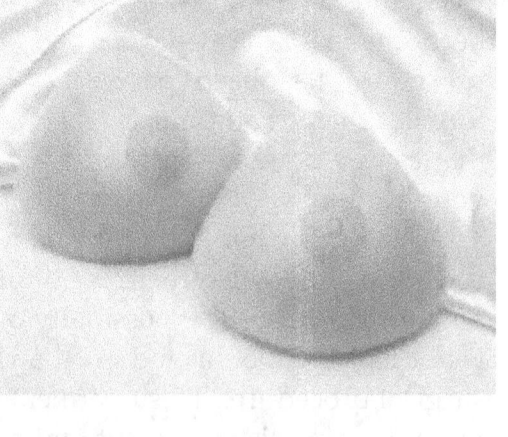

tions relating to the breast removal procedure. The problem can be fixed, by removing the cause and not the breast(s). It's very important for you to understand the difference, which can mean keeping a breast or two.

The proper defense can be looked at in two senses; *from*

and *out of.* First, to protect women *from* "re-construction" --- keeping them from entering into it; and secondly, if they have already entered it, to provide comfort and relief efforts *out of* it. The first safeguard would be most precious to millions; the second is an offer to numerous victims.

In the medical profession, there are two features of breast removal to be considered; cut first and ask questions later. Women all over the world are being cut open for all the wrong reasons. It is every woman's nightmare – for good reason. The results are a reconstructed breast, made up of a silicone bag filled with a saline solution; a prosthetic bra with a prosthesis; topped off with a wig and a lymphadema sleeve and glove which helps reduce swelling of the arm and hands. This is what the average woman encounters after breast removal surgery. Some women that opt for this surgical procedure think long and hard before deciding to go forward with it. You may have been one of those individuals or you know of family and friends who have gone through this affair.

Another way to look at breast cancer or other breast disorders is that the breasts are under assault. Typically, when something is attacked, a shield of protection is needed. Painfully, many are "unlearning" all the myths that involve breast cancer. It is not all its cut out to be.

As stated earlier, breast cancer is a process. To many it's a painful process. What takes place, from beginning to end, varies with each individual. One variation to look at happens like this: when a cancerous tumor is found in the breast, at the advice of a physician, along with encouragement and support from family and friends, most women usually consent to the following sequence of events:

1. Biopsy, and

2.  Lumpectomy (surgical removal of the tumor) or
3.  Mastectomy (surgical removal of the breast) with removal of some of the (underarm) lymph nodes; plus
4.  Radiation therapy, chemotherapy (before or after hormone therapy (drugs) and/or
5.  Double Mastectomy (surgical removal of other breast)

After some or all of these treatments, the current medical paradigm is relatively clueless about what causes breast cancer and how to effectively treat it. Most conventional cancer treatments actually add insult to injury by doing more harm than good — a fact that up to this point has been swept under the rug by the medical industry.

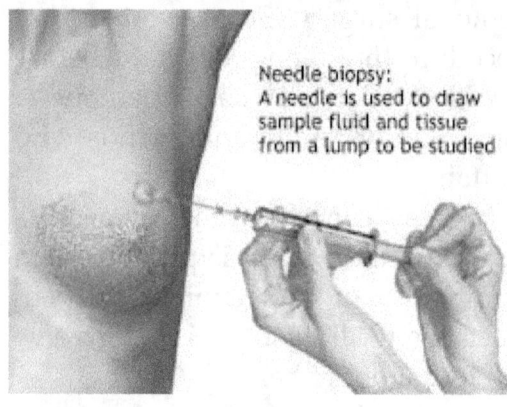

Needle biopsy:
A needle is used to draw sample fluid and tissue from a lump to be studied

I hope you are starting to see that the medical establishment is seriously on the wrong track where breast cancer is concerned. Some women have embraced a collapsing system of successively more intense, unneeded interventions termed "standard of care." A seemingly healthy woman with nothing more than a tiny lump in her breast could agree to have a biopsy performed not knowing whether she would awake from surgery with a small bandage on her breast -- or no breast at all. This system needs changing.

When a woman experiences sensations and reactions in her breasts, nature is speaking. Do not overlook its role or ignore its warning signals. I Corinthians 11:14 says *"Doth not even nature itself teach you.....?"* Nature provides everything we need to gain and defend a good condition of health. The varied wonders of nature speak through the body which is beyond human comprehension.

For example, we live in an orderly universe that is subject to the law of cause and effect. If you throw a ball up in the air, the law of gravity will make it come back down. If it doesn't, there is a reason. This law is also true of our health. It is sometimes hard to see the cause and effect connection between the health laws and the consequences of disregarding them, simply because the effects are not immediate. Therefore, to reason from cause to effect, enlightened by understanding, must hold the reins of influence.

Consider briefly, when a woman's breast is removed, it affects some other part of the body disabling it to do its proper share of the work. In essence, some other organ takes on the extra work. In a normal condition, there is harmonious action of all the members of the body and mind that results in a pleasant feeling of health.

Danger is often the means whereby deliverance comes to a person with an illness or disease, many not realizing that your predicament has been the means of delivering you from far greater evil. No evil can be warded off unless it is first recognized. In nature, the fox hides to its hole for protection; the bird flies to the wood for shelter; and even so the breast-stricken woman hastens to someone or something for safety. Normally, it's the former rather than the latter.

Many breast cancer reconstructions and deaths are preventable, and a good share of the blame for these horrific ordeals and fatalities may be attributed to the unfortunate women, along with their health care providers. A best kept secret, not revealed or known by doctors, is that the body was built with safeguards and healing powers within. For example, when we are cut, the body starts to work trying to repair the damage. When we are invaded by a sickness or disease, the body's immune system is alerted and starts to defend against the illness. In most cases of breast cancer, women are the ones that notice something's wrong of the breasts that don't look or feel right.

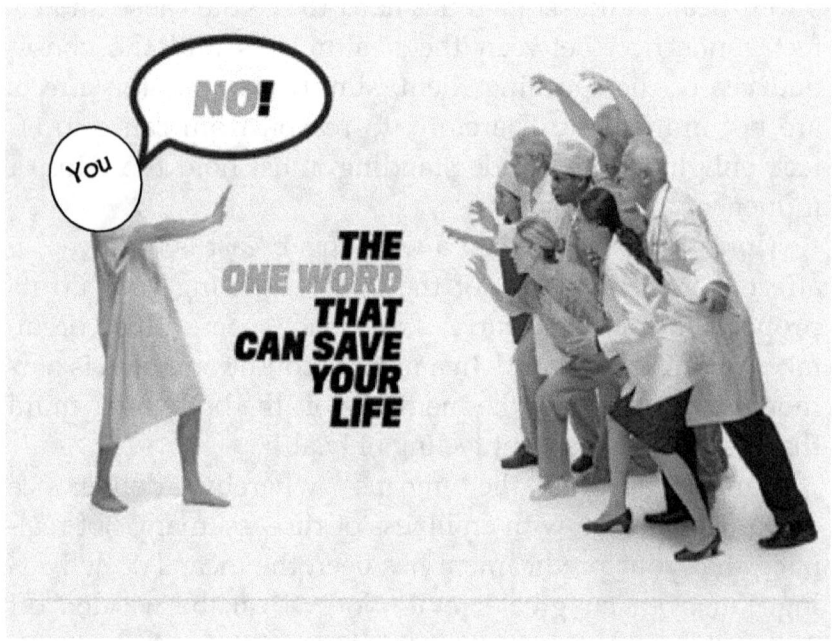

In the past, the old-fashioned approach to most diseases dealt with finding the cause. At present, the medical community has created a world of specialists and compartmentalized the body. If the illness deals with a female, first you go to your ob/gyn. If cancer is found, then you are sent to the oncologist. Therefore, in this scenario, breast cancer is sent through the system. If anyone has been watching the media, they know that there are problems with the medical systems. Big problems!

This thought brings us to the medical profession that prides themselves on being "scientific." I believe that work is called "science." When it comes to the body, what is science? I believe that the following paragraph beautifully depicts the meaning of science:

> **"All true science is but an interpretation of the handwriting of God in the material world. Science brings from her research only fresh evidences of the wisdom and power of God. Rightly understood, both the book of nature and the written word make us acquainted with God by teaching us something of the wise and beneficent laws through which he works."** *Counsels on Health, p. 66.*

Based on this passage, conventional medicine is not very scientific. Today, science is seeking for truth. God's Word is truth (see John 17:17) and while science changes it theories and even its "facts" with the passing years, God's Word remains.

In addition, many women are frustrated with orthodox medicine and are aggressively seeking information and new choices for their healthcare, especially for breast cancer. More and more women are learning to weigh their actions, measuring the loss and gain, removing any self-indulgent purposes, and devoting to doing the right things to be in health. In doing this, it sends the message that the breasts are not the cause of their cancer, but only the "housing" of the effect!

When it comes to surgical procedures, the answer is often no. No studies prove that procedures like a radical mastectomy (breast removal) are beneficial to the female. Instead, there are studies that show they *don't* work and most times are detrimental to the woman's health.     Undeservingly, this procedure is given wide publicity.

As a matter of fact, during the editing of this book, a news story hot off the press (May, 2013) reported that Angelina Jolie had just underwent a double mastectomy. The timing could not have been better. Why? Because since this story surfaced, many women have opted to follow the footsteps of this "movie star" who is portrayed as one of Hollywood's beauty figure on television and entertainment magazines. Here is a reprint of that story for your perusal:

*(CNN) -- Actress Angelina Jolie announced in a New York Times op-ed article on Tuesday that she underwent a preventive double mastectomy after learning that she carries a mutation of the BRCA1 gene, which sharply increases her risk of developing breast cancer and ovarian cancer.*

*"My doctors estimated that I had an 87 percent risk of breast cancer and a 50 percent risk of ovarian cancer, although the risk is different in the case of each woman," Jolie wrote. "Once I knew that this was my reality, I decided to be proactive and to minimize the risk as much I could. I made a decision to have a preventive double mastectomy."*

*She wrote that her experience involved a three-step process. On February 2, the actress had a procedure that increases the chance that the nipple can be saved. Two weeks later, she had major surgery where the breast tissue was removed and temporary fillers were put in place. Nine weeks later, she described undergoing "reconstruction of the breasts with an implant.     In telling her story, Jolie acknowledged that surgery might not be the right choice for every woman.*

*"For any woman reading this, I hope it helps you to know you have options," Jolie wrote. "I want to encourage every woman, especially if you have a family history of breast or ovarian cancer, to seek out the information and medical experts who can help you through this aspect of your life, and to make your own informed choices."*

Making GOOD choices is, without a doubt, a "Life's Work!" It's not something you do for a few days – and then you're done! Being a woman -- wife, daughter, sister, mother-- requires the hard task of making good choices during their lifetime. Few are willing to consistently pay the price required.

Consider this scenario. After receiving a breast cancer diagnosis, most women are afraid and even frantic to do whatever it takes, as soon as possible, to fight and remove the cancer. And usually, that involves the "slash and burn" approach. Can you imagine what it would be like to go through surgery, having one or both of your breasts re-moved along with receiving debilitating radiation treat-ments and toxic drugs, only to later be told that you *never had cancer*?

This scenario happens more often than you might think. If you don't believe it happens, "Google it" on the internet and witness the terrifying ordeals women experience with false breast cancer diagnoses.

On the other hand, the Bible warns us about what hap-pens when we make poor choices as follows:

*"There is a way that seemeth right unto a man, but the end thereof [are] the ways of death."* (Proverbs 16:25).

*"[It is] better to trust in the LORD than to put confidence in man."* (Psalms 118:8).

*"Thus saith the LORD; Cursed [be] the man that trusteth in man, and maketh flesh his arm,.."* (Jeremiah 17:5).

If you get nothing else out of this book, I want you to get this: Your responsibility regarding your own health is very important. You are the most important member of your "medical team." You have been given the freedom of choice regarding your health. To place in the hands of any human being the power to dominate your thinking, either by surgery or other means, is to create a situation laden with the gravest danger.

Doing what's right takes dedication, determination and a great deal of prayer. Satan knows that destroying the woman is paramount in his plan to destroy the individual. He makes the wide road very tempting when it comes to making 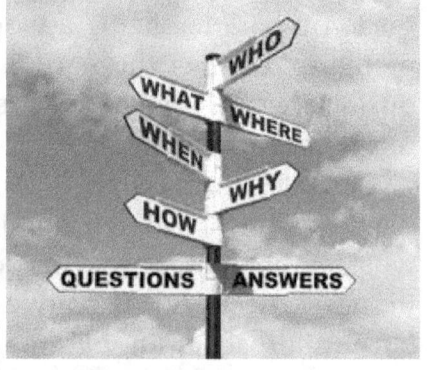 "choices." Hence, we must make sure that all of our choices are "<u>right</u>eous" ones. Pray for wisdom in all that you do, especially regarding your breasts!

You see, while knowledge is powerful, it boils down to your attitude towards your breasts. Do you expect good or bad things? Success or failure? Victory or defeat? Will you be a "victim" or "victor?"

If you are serious about keeping your breasts, a commitment is necessary and specific changes must be made. The very fact that you have made it thus far to this point of the book, it's a good indication that you are! If you have breast cancer or one of the other breast disorders, stay positive and know that there is light at the end of the long, hard tunnel. By faith, you will get through this, and come out on the other end feeling like a well-informed and stronger person.

# Chapter 6

## Breast Care: Prevention and Cure

*Routine.   Privilege.   Natural.*

Upon you who have been given breasts, there rests a great responsibility that, if accepted seriously and carried out intelligently, brings reward beyond compare. Women, to your breasts you owe a sound development and a disease-free environment. The achievement of each of these depends upon you. Your reward is the untold happiness derived from a common-sense attitude about your breasts and a future free from those conditions that result in breast cancer and other breast disorders. This section is written with the hope that it will provide a plateau for women to view their current breasts health practices – and step more vigorously into a healthier mindset towards them.

In today's society, great care is provided for almost all parts of the body – hair, nails, feet, face, teeth, eyes, and the list goes on. Personalized care is very personal -- if not for correction, for the sake of appearance. Proper breast care, when expanded over the years of a woman's life, is not only a *beginning* in the ways of health, but also a *continuance* in the same as long as life lasts. Not only is proper breast care extremely important and highly invaluable, it is a woman's privilege.

In the highest sense, it should become a woman's study to become intimately acquainted with her breasts. Taking the time to give full attention to them is one of the most important things you can do. No one can take care of your breasts better than you. Everything starts with 'care' which requires diligent effort.

Although proper breast care is a natural procedure, it doesn't come naturally to every woman. If never taught, it's a learning experience. As you put your breasts forward, it is important to keep track of them for health reasons. There still remains today too many women who believe that once their breasts are developed, their health is already determined and that whatever happens during their lifetime is unimportant to the well-being of them. This idea is not justified. By doing their part, it is up to each woman, to see that their breasts receive the maximum care and be kept in health.

Every October, in America, a big to-do is made about breast cancer. It is called National Breast Cancer Awareness month. With pink ribbons and rally marches, this time

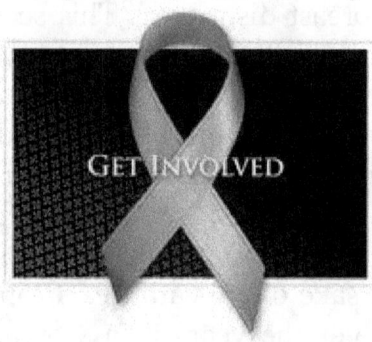

is dedicated to increasing awareness about the importance of the early detection of breast cancer. Why? Around the clock, a woman is diagnosed with breast cancer.

Unfortunately, breast cancer is not bound by a particular month. Its occurrence can happen at anytime. Undeniably, early detection is good in itself but the main thrust of this campaign should be breast cancer prevention.

An old adage that has been stressed with repetition regarding health is *"An ounce of prevention is worth a pound of cure."* No important truth has been more concisely stated or more effective, if heeded. On the contrary, this important principle has almost gone amiss today. Instead, it appears that this present saying has become the norm; *"It's my body and I do what I want to with it!"*

The gospel of prevention is a breast-saving message. How? It provides a means to avoid disorders and deficiencies that may prove injurious to you – especially your breasts. To a great degree, if women would be more health-wise, they would enter into the experience that's often talked about but seldom realized as spoken of in 3 John 2, *"Beloved, I wish above all things that thou prosper and be in health, so that thy soul may prosper."*

Briefly, let's focus on women who rely on other entities to care for their breasts. When breast cancer is suspected, doctors are urged to "do something" to figure out what's wrong. Often doctors feel that the way to demonstrate that they are doing something is to order tests. Since cancer spreads in the body through the lymph system and through the blood, to determine how far the breast cancer has spread, doctors will order a series of imaging tests. Among the many ways Americans are over-tested, imaging is one of the most common. Many fret about airport scanners, power lines, cell phones and even microwaves. It is true that they give off **too much radiation**. But it's not only from those sources. It's from the recommended medical tests -- like mammograms.

With this in mind, at one time, women who turned 40 were encouraged to start getting annual mammograms for early detection. However, a controversy over screening mammography flared up in 2009, when a government funded group of independent experts decided to change its recommendations. Instead of advising annual mammograms in all women at age 40, the U.S. Preventive Services Task Force (USPSTF) said women shouldn't routinely get screened until age 50, and those between 50 and 74 should only have mammograms every two years.   Long 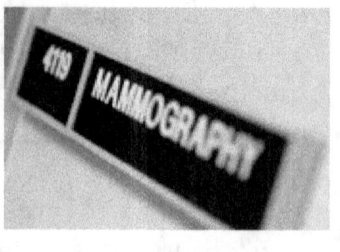 story short, advocacy groups, news organizations, and medical groups protested.  In essence, they felt the new guidelines were unsafe.

Women who favor mammograms, I submit the following evidences to support the topic under investigation.  It has been reported that doctors don't keep track of radiation given their patients — they order a test, not a dose.  Radiation is a hidden danger, although with mammograms, there are federal rules prohibiting too much radiation dose. Mammograms expose your body to radiation that can be 1,000 times greater than a chest x-ray, which we know poses a cancer risk.   It is well known that ionizing radiation increases the cellular mutations that lead to cancer — and mammograms aim a highly focused dose directly at your breasts, thereby increasing your cancer risk!  WHY would you want to do this?

Mammography also compresses your breasts tightly, and often painfully, which could lead to a lethal spread of cancerous cells, should they exist. Dr. Charles B. Simone, a former clinical associate in immunology and pharmacology at the National Cancer Institute, said: "*Mammograms increase the risk for developing breast cancer and raise the risk of spreading or metastasizing an existing growth.*"

In July 1995,  an article in **_The Lancet_** about mammograms read:  "*The benefit is marginal, the harm caused is substantial, and the costs incurred are enormous.*"  There is no solid evidence that mammograms save lives, in spite of the propaganda some organizations constantly mimic to the press. Mammograms are often flaunted as a "life-saving" form of cancer screening, responsible for reducing breast cancer death rates by 15 to 25 percent. But this reported benefit is based on outdated studies done *decades* ago.

First of its kind, a recent study was published in the *New England Journal of Medicine,* (September, 2010) to look at the effectiveness of mammograms. This prominent medical journals' findings are a far cry from what most public health officials and physicians would have you believe. The study showed that mammograms might have only reduced cancer death rates by 0.4 deaths per 1,000 women — an amount so small it may as well be zero. To put it another way, 2,500 women would have to be screened over 10 years for a single breast cancer death to be avoided.

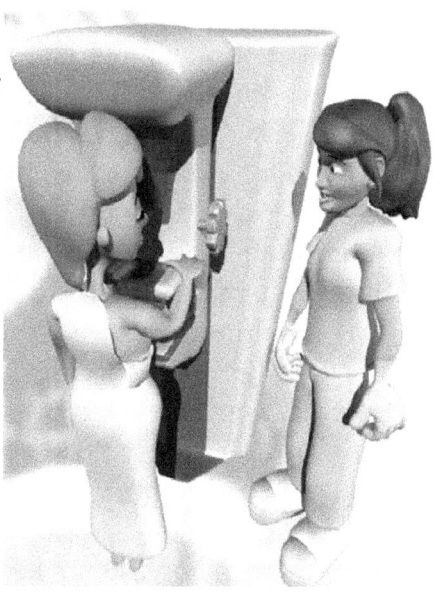

So, not only are mammograms unsafe, but they are NOT saving lives as many medical professionals believed they were. Past research has also demonstrated that adding an annual mammogram to a physical examination of the breasts does not improve breast cancer survival rates either.

Another featured problem with mammography is its **unacceptably high rate of false positives**. If a mammogram detects an abnormal spot in a woman's breast, the next step is typically a biopsy. This involves taking a small amount of tissue from the breast, which is then looked at by a pathologist under a microscope to determine if cancer is present. Estimates are that 17 percent of DCIS cases found through needle biopsy are misdiagnosed.

False positives can lead to unnecessary emotional stress and expensive repeat screenings, exposing you to even more radiation, chemotherapy, and unnecessary invasive procedures including biopsies and major surgery. Women have actually undergone **unnecessary mastectomies** after receiving a false positive mammogram report.

Whatever position you hold concerning this matter, the next time the thought or suggestion comes to you about getting a mammogram, put these reasons in your decision-making memory bank:

- Mammograms are largely useless.
- Women end up being unnecessarily treated for a disease they do not have.
- Mammograms actually <u>increase</u> women's **risk** of getting breast cancer.
- Dense breasts make routine mammograms difficult to read.
- The vast majority of tumors detected by mammography are not even malignant, which often leads to costly and unnecessary interventions.
- Mammograms produce faulty and false findings.
- Latest study shows that mammograms will not prevent you from getting breast cancer.

The final analysis of the benefits of mammography is -- early detection is only as good as the treatments that follow. Then the question is, after getting a mammogram, how many lives will be saved by surgery, radiation, chemotherapy, or hormone treatment? If your answer is not many, you may want to consider skipping the next mammogram based on this --it can do more harm than good. Actually, mammograms will not *prevent you* from getting breast cancer, and the latest study shows they offer very little benefit in improving your chances of survival. Effective cancer preventing methods are important, but mammography is simply NOT the answer.

To me, it appears that mammograms have become a crutch for doctors. How? By not using breast exams and sound judgment decisions to make a diagnosis. Oops, I forgot. In medical school, doctors are not taught to make sound judgment evaluations. Instead, their ideology is to medicate or operate. Then, what is the answer?

Alternatively, breast self-exams have long been recommended as a simple way for women to keep track of anything unusual in their breasts. Now, after studies have found that such exams do not reduce breast cancer death rates and actually increase the rate of unnecessary biopsies, many experts are recommending a more relaxed approach known as "**breast awareness**."

Breast awareness is really self-explanatory. It means you should regularly check your breasts for changes, but can do so in a way that feels natural to you. In other words, you don't have to do it on the same day each month, or using any particular pattern. Simply be aware of what's normal for you so you can recognize anything out of the ordinary. Although breast cancer is much less common in men, it certainly wouldn't hurt for men to practice "breast awareness" as well.

Are we offering a technique or instructions on how to do monthly self-exams? No, but appealing to women to be more alert to how their breasts look and feel in general so they can detect any noticeable changes.

Not to miss the essential message of breast care, one must understand that the how it's done is as important as, if not more important than, what is done. Breast care, even though exercised reasonably, can be carried to excess. What's needed is a good working knowledge that will make you feel a lot more secure --and a lot less nervous.

Knowledge is power. It can take just one tidbit of information to prevent disease or even save a life. Making that knowledge a guide in life empowers you to take more responsibility for your breast health. However, this may require you to reverse a few practices you thought were beneficial, and make what you consider substantial sacrifices in your lifestyle. This all translates into an opportunity to take control of your breasts, rather than leave them in the hands of destiny or someone else.

Most, if not all, of the deaths from breast cancer can be prevented by proper attention and care and by skillful remedial methods. In reality, breast care begins at the time of birth. To help avoid any risks during infancy to adolescent years, the ideal arrangement is for a mother or guardian to have the thorough knowledge themselves to impart it to their daughters or relatives alike.

As young girls advance in years, instruction in this line should be continued until they are qualified to care for themselves. For the most part, young women don't consider breast care as important now. It's something that lurks in the distant future, sometimes 20 to 30 years away. The overall goal is to have them understand the importance of preserving the vitality of the breasts to guard against disease, and to inform their mother/guardian when something appears unusual or wrong to them. Many adults, who did not learn this lesson, early in life, are now exhibiting lifelong health problems as a result.

Stay on top of your breasts. Do what it takes – to keep your breasts under your jurisdiction. You can have the mastery over them, if you conscientiously strive to fulfill your part. Everything you choose to do, or not do, will either bring health and well-being or disease and misery. The value of proper breast care stresses intelligent supervision and prevention methods. Such care is absolutely necessary and helpful for all women. No other preventative way offers such remarkable returns in sparing the breasts from suffering disease.

To embrace an effective model of breast care, women (i.e. mothers, grandmothers, teenagers) must educate themselves to the true process of taking care of the body. Pay attention to your breasts. To keep track of them doesn't require keeping a journal or dissecting them. The key is finding a method that works for you.

A healthy, familiar routine that is established early in life can be beneficial for a lifetime. Familiarize your breasts with routine care. It does the breasts well. Let your sense of sight and touch guide you. Hence, as a breast initiative, make it a routine task of checking and inspecting them. Being familiar with each breasts' size and shape lets you discern change, if any. You'll notice them more than anyone else, because you're looking down or at them. Along with this initiative, you might want to keep breast notes (in the "Write" Things section). They can serve as reminders that keep you attentive, responsive and attuned to your breasts. Remember, the breasts are within your own reach. If you don't get to them, they will eventually get to you.

As you become better acquainted with your breasts,

your mind will become more educated. Your skill at interpreting your own breasts' language will improve with practice; in the meantime, every woman should naturally look for clues to the breasts needs. These clues will help direct you on what to do for your breasts, whether you should continue what you've been doing, try something different or simply stand back and observe them. You can protect your breasts from all the struggles they might go through in life.

Thousands of women fail to do the things necessary to prevent breast disease because of ignorance, negligence, financial difficulties or other reasons. Consequently, they neglect to carry out specific practices that are of the utmost importance to their own health. In this world of ours nothing that is truly worth possessing is attained without persevering efforts and untiring attention. You must regain faith in knowing the body and look what it is telling you. In short, we must be on watch of our own health.

At this point, it seems well to consider what the Bible has to say about the entire subject of your body, especially since little or no dealing with Biblical background is found in breast cancer material published. A good passage to begin with is found in Proverbs 4:20-22: *"My son (daughter), attend to my words; incline thine ear unto my sayings. Let them not depart from thine eyes; keep them in the midst of thine heart. For they [are] life unto those that find them, and health to all their flesh."* If we attend to God's words, they are life, and health is promised. Another way to say it is, we must follow God's health laws. They protect the body against severe conditions and share in the care of the breasts. Each one contains simple instructions and principles that should be followed in the daily life.

Getting down to business about preserving your health

is all about one's use of time. But time has a tendency of slipping through our fingers – and you must learn to snatch it back. Therefore, to help you harness your time and get busy with your breasts, we've incorporated these health laws into an acronym --- A.B.R.E.A.S.T.S. to keep you well informed.

A.B.R.E.A.S.T.S. represent a compilation of all the general principles of health preservation and restoration that cause the body, and help the breast, to be restored to health. Those who fail to observe them can-not hope to regain health or even to maintain it at its present level. Not one female who complies with these health laws will be disappointed in the end; not one who is earnest and desires to succeed will fail. If you don't apply them to your life-style daily, it's guaranteed the breasts will be affected.

**A.**lign with God
**B.**reath of Life
**R.**efreshing Water
**E.**ating Properly
**A.**ctive Exercise
**S.**leep and Rest
**T.**emperance Messengers
**S**unshine Rays

**Align with God:** *"There are thousands, yes, millions, who are making a mistake in their religious life. They make re-ligion a thing independent of their life, or their thoughts and words, and daily actions."* The Signs of the Time, Feb-ruary 28, 1895.

Commune with God daily –morning and evening. God's promises in the Bible are the means by which we place our trust in Him. Eliminate stress...and put God to the test.

**Scripture References:**
    Isaiah 26:4        Psalms 5:1-3
    Matthew 11:29-30    I Peter 5:7

**Breath of Life:** *"The health of the entire system depends upon the healthy action of the respiratory organs."* Healthful Living, p. 30.

Spend time outdoors and breathe deeply. Breathing through your nose when you inhale, your stomach should go out. When you exhale, your stomach should go in. Sleep with windows cracked throughout year for proper ventilation. Pray every day for it is the breath of the soul.

**Scripture References:**
    Job 33:4        Philippians 2:15, 16
    Acts 26:18      1 John 1:5

**Refreshing Water:** *"Thousands have died for want of pure water...who might have lived...These blessings they need in order to become well..."* Counsels on Diet and Food, p. 419

Drink water by measure daily, from time to time. To determine your water intake, divide your body weight by 2. This is the number of ounces of water you should drink every day. Avoid liquid counterfeits i.e., tea, coffee, alcohol, sodas that are poisonous to the system. Frequent cleansing of the body helps rid the body of impurities.

**Scripture references:**

Revelation 21:6      Psalms 51:7, 9
Ezekiel 4:11      I Timothy 5:23
Proverbs 20:1

**Eating Properly:** *"There are few who realize as they should how much their habits of diet have to do with their health..."* Patriarchs and Prophets, p. 562.

Fruits, vegetables, nuts, and whole grains are helpful in maintaining good health. Avoid these foods: all soft drinks, coffee and tea, condiments, spices, white/brown sugar, meats (fish, chicken, etc.) dairy products, refined and processed foods, fried foods, can foods. Eliminate eating between meals (allow at least 5 hours) or late at night (allow 3 hours before bedtime).

**Scripture references:**

Genesis 1:28-29      Genesis 3:18
Proverbs 23:3      1 Corinthians 10:31

**Active Exercise:** *"Inactivity is a fruitful cause of disease. Exercise quickens and equalizes the circulation of the blood."* My Life Today, p. 130.

Exercise should be consistent. It should be vigorous enough to maintain a sustained increase heart rate. If immobile, a massage is recommended. Outdoor is best. Walking and gardening are perfect for this purpose. For spiritual exercise, dwell upon the things of God and study His Word. Involvement in proper recreation is highly beneficial to both mind and body.

**Scripture references:**

Psalms 128:2          Mark 6:31

Luke 12:30, 31        Genesis 2:8, 15

**Sleep and Rest:** *"Sleep, nature's sweet restorer, invigorates the weary body and prepares it for the next day's duties."* The Adventist Home, p. 289.

A pattern or a regular bedtime and arising time, without weekend or seasonal variations, should be the order of life. Go to bed and wake up at regular times every day. For sleeping, make it an "early to bed, early to rise" habit. To rest is just not to sleep. Take times of relaxation to be refreshed physically, mentally, and spiritually. Experience a weekly blessing by resting on the seventh day.

**Scripture references:**

Matthew 11:28       Psalms 104:20-23

Exodus 20:8-11      Hebrews 4:11, 16

**Temperance Messengers**: *"A pure and noble life, a life of victory over appetite and lust, is possible to everyone"* The Faith I Live By, p. 154.

Do not overwork, overeat, or under dress. Regularity in all things is essential. Keeping the appetite under control, keeps the body in subjection. What you permit in your life, you promote.

**Scripture references:**

Romans 12:1        I Corinthians 3:17

Isaiah 6:10

**Sunlight Rays:** *"The sun is a God-given physician."*
Manuscript Releases, vol. 20, p. 25.

Exposure to your hands and face are essential. Properly used, sunshine is a great light that kills bacteria, provides vitamin D, and gives off warmth and beauty. It's free to all and one of heaven's blessings.

**Scripture references:**

| | |
|---|---|
| Malachi 4:2 | Genesis 1:16 |
| Matthew 5:45 | Ecclesiastes 11:7 |

Breast cancer and other breast disorders are preventable. But if you are hit with that diagnosis, don't lose hope! There is a great deal you can do to harness your body's own powerful healing abilities. And the good news is that with information, resources and the will to change your lifestyle, you can make the necessary changes to ensure that you live a long and healthy life.

Keep in mind, if you are diagnosed with breast cancer, and you find it necessary to go the medical way, please get a second—and possibly third and fourth—opinion. I cannot stress this enough, since the false positive rates are just too high and the diagnostic criteria too subjective.

Moreover, before you make any decision on treatment—and definitely before you decide to have surgery or chemotherapy—make sure your biopsy results have been reviewed by the 'best breast specialist" who is knowledgeable and experienced in that field. That individual is none other than Jesus Christ. Don't' forget to take all your diagnosis to Him. Furthermore, let him be your "Physician." He's NUMBER ONE IN ALL FIELDS.

Ladies, adopt a healthy attitude toward your breasts because the years of life will slip by quickly. Whatever state your health is in — prevention or cure — always keep abreast. Not only will your breasts benefit, but your entire body will too. It's time to get down to business!

## Chapter 7

*Not By Prescription*

*Power.   Restore.   Triumph.*

The clarion call has gone out. Breast health is worth embracing and celebrating.   Good health is worth more than money in the bank.   With all the information shared in this book, we come full circle to the title *"Keeping A-Breast or Two"* – the practical side of how to.   This section is where the rubber hits the road, so to speak. It is for those who are ready to 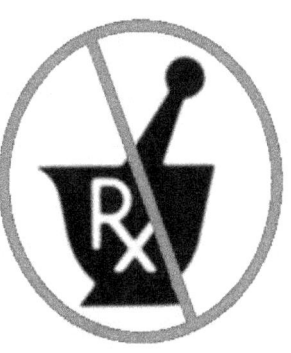 raise their commitment to health.   The access road to "the remedy" has lead us to this chapter.

There are three filters that set "the remedy" for breast cancer and other breast disorders apart from every other healing philosophies.   First, the remedy is found in the written Word of God.   It begins and ends here.   God has given us simple directions.   Carefully followed, God's written instruction is indeed *"no vain thing for you, because it is your life:...ye shall prolong your days in the land..."* (Deuteronomy. 32:47).

Additionally, it is not founded on meditation or whim; not obtainable by swishing some secret potent around in your mouth; not rooted in video hypnosis or an emotional high; the remedy is simply living out the written instructions given by God.   This very simplicity is what gives it power.

Secondly, "the remedy" requires a lifestyle change. In the knowledge and power of God alone can health-destroying habits be broken. Only in Christ is there motive and strength enough to break the bondage of long-established habits. Lifestyle changes are quite possible without Christ, but that transformation which makes a person whole (healed) is not. Only in the belief in a loving God and an all-wise Father can we achieve that totally changed lifestyle that leads to total health.

Lastly, "the remedy" calls for self-denial that has purpose and sense. Everyone will make a sacrifice; but few deny self in the way God knows will be effective. Self-indulgence is the order of these days. Have you heard this saying before — *"Health is desired by many, but chosen by few."* This should be alarming, but it is not. Straightforwardly, *"to have health, you must live for it!"*

For those who suffer from breast disease (cancer) and the rest of the indulgence-produced maladies, self-denial is at the heart of "the remedy." To deny self is simply to do what God asks. Deny self of the S.A.D.; deny self of the stressors; deny self of the unhealthy dress. In the power of Christ, deny self of **all** that would destroy your health.

If you are like the woman spoken about in Matthew 9:21, who spent her means on physicians, treatments, and prescription drugs, only to still be pronounced incurable, you may or may not know what was required of her to be healed. Simply, faith! Without doubt, faith is the driving force of "the remedy," determining the outcome and making your healing experience inestimable.

If you want access to this kind of healing, ask the "Great Physician." The Great Physician here referred to is Jesus, the Son of God. He has all the "true" prescriptions for the diseases that plague women and millions alike today.

The scripture states that it is *"The Lord who forgiveth all thine iniquities; who healeth all thy diseases."* (Psalms 103: 5). The good news is that these prescriptions are available to all people; user friendly; inexpensive; simple to understand; and have no adverse side effects. In their totality, they are effective, invaluable, highly profound, and brings peace, joy and health.

In regard to that which we can do for ourselves, it would be beneficial to consider these words based on John 11:39, *"Take ye away the stone."*

**"Christ could have commanded the stone to be removed, and it would have obeyed His voice. He could have bidden the angels who were close by His side to do this. At His bidding, invisible hands would have removed the stone. But it was to be taken away by human hands. Thus Christ would show that humanity is to co-operate with divinity. What human power can do divine power is not summoned to do. God does not dispense with man's aid. He strengthens him, co-operating with him as he uses the powers and capabilities given him."** *Desire of Ages, p.535.*

Along with the eight laws of health — A.B.R.E.A.S.T.S. (chapter 6), there are many natural remedies which will do much to restore the breasts back to health. Some require simple preparations and others may require assistance. However, to those who reach out to God to direct them, is the time when divine help is nearest. Remember, only you can decide what to try to help you achieve having healthy breasts.

## THE REMEDY

When you think of breast disease, think of a mountain. If you want it to go away, you need to implement the mustard seed mountain moving principle that Jesus taught in Matthew 17:20-21. The first step in moving the mountain of breast disease, or any other mountains in your life is to have faith and obey. You must alleviate stress, bombard the body with nutrition, equalize circulation, and cleanse the system. The only way to accomplish these is to apply *God's Healing Way!*

**APPROACH:**  The rational plan of treatment for "breast cancer requires first, the removal of the causes by which the condition has been produced, if and when they are still in operation; secondly, bring relief  to the breasts by proper treatment; thirdly, alleviation of the symptoms attending this  condition; fourth, restoration of the breasts to a healthy condition.

All breast diseases can be removed by the individual's faithful and diligent implementation of the following:

<u>**PROTOCOL**</u>
 Daily application  of the following is  necessary to facilitate healing.
- 8 laws of health (refer to chapter 6)
- Herbal Therapy
- Dietary Therapy
- Hydrotherapy

A cleanse  should be undertaken for  7 or 10 days depending upon the severity of the case and upon the tolerance of the individual..   The more days… the healthier. During this time, nothing should be taken but the juices of fruits and vegetables (low estrogen foods, if applicable).
 Juicing of vegetables is very beneficial. The drink should

be made palatable so the patient may take copious amounts may be added to the juice.   A juice fast also normalizes and corrects most other disturbances and malfunctions in the body which might be contributing causes to the disease.

Through the process of breathing, oxygen is taken into the system. This oxygen combines with the waste matter to form carbon dioxide. If we do not get rid of this waste matter, nature increases the blood pressure to force the blood to the lungs to absorb more oxygen.  In order to assist nature in her attempt to correct this condition, we must first help her in her task of cleansing the body of waste deposits.

Every night of the fast, an enema or colonic, consisting of warm water and garlic water should be used to cleanse the body of the poisons and wastes which are being loosened by the action of the juices.

**Lemon Water** – Drink the juice of ½ lemon or lime freshly squeezed in 14 oz. of warm water. **(Take first thing in morning upon rising).**

When we cleanse the body, it  builds up good healthy cells which can do their work of keeping the body functioning properly.

It will  be  astonishing to most people to note the results they will  obtain in  this  length of  time,  but it is simply a matter of cooperating with the body and assisting, instead of hindering its effort to help the body heal itself.

\*\*\*\*\*\*\*\*\*\*\*\*\*\*\*\*\*\*\*\*\*\*\*\*\*\*\*\*\*\*\*\*\*\*\*\*\*\*\*\*\*\*\*\*\*\*\*\*

## DIETARY CONSIDERATIONS:

**Juice Diet:** Use any combination of the following vegetables:   Broccoli, kale, turnip greens, beets, carrots   (limit ounces if high estrogen cancer).  Mix and drink 16 ounces, 3 times daily.

After the fast, the diet should consist of nothing but raw fruits and vegetables for at least two to three months.   No starch, fat, or protein whatsoever should be taken during this period.

After the restricted diet, other things may be added the diet consisting of the following: Fruits and vegetables, both raw and cooked, raw fruit juices, raw vegetable juices in generous amounts and, whole grain: bread and cereals.

Salad Dressing (opt.) Mix 2 Tbsp lemon juice, 2 Tbsp olive oil, 1 Tbsp honey, herb seasoning to taste.  Emphasis on low estrogen foods (if applicable).

## LOW ESTROGEN FOODS

| | |
|---|---|
| *Quinoa | * Figs |
| *Millet | * All Melons |
| *Kamut | * Peaches |
| *Aramanth | * Pears |
| *Honey | * Oranges |
| * Radishes | * Mangoes |
| * Kale | * Lemons |
| * Cabbage | * Raisins |
| * Brussels Sprouts | * Apricots |
| * Turnips | * Grapefruits |
| * Beets | * Prunes |
| * Mustard Greens | * Grapes |
| * Lettuce | * Strawberries |
| * Spinach | * Blue/Blackberries |
| * Celery | * Thyme |
| * Broccoli | * Squash |

* Cauliflower
* Fresh Peas
* String Beans
* Flax Seeds
* Sunflower Seeds
* Sesame Seeds
* Flax Seeds

* Okra
* Cucumbers
* Pumpkin

\*\*\*\*\*\*\*\*\*\*\*\*\*\*\*\*\*\*\*\*\*\*\*\*\*\*\*\*\*\*\*\*\*\*\*\*\*\*\*\*\*\*\*\*\*\*\*\*\*\*\*\*\*

## HERBAL CONSIDERATIONS:

This formula consists of immune enhancing, tumor reducing herbs  that can be used to shrink any tumors.

**Herbal Mixture**

| | |
|---|---|
| Astragalus | 3 parts |
| Chaparral | 2 parts |
| Red Raspberry | 2 parts |
| Echinacea | 5 parts |
| Pau D Arco | 3 parts |
| Red Clover | 5 parts |
| Chlorella or Spirulina | 3 parts |
| Or any green food | |

Mix all together to make a tea using 2 TBSP in  one  cup of hot  water (let steep for 20 min). Drink three times daily. You can take these herbs as teas or as capsules or tinctures depending on the availability of the herbs in your locality.

## COLON CLEANSING DRINK

This formula is an herbal (powder) colon cleanser.  It consists of  Psyllium  Husk  (3  parts) ,  Slippery  Elm  (2  parts),

Cayenne Pepper (1/16 part), Bentonite Clay or Mandrake ( 1 part), Senna  or Cascara Sagrada (1 part), and Apple Pectin (2 parts), Wormwood or Black walnut (1 part), Activated Charcoal (1 part).  Mix in a bowl and store in glass jar.

Place one heaping Tbsp. of the Colon Cleanser Formula into a  jar with a lid and add about 4 — 6 oz. of fruit apple or grape juice. **If diabetic**, use 4 oz. of water instead of the fruit juice.  Shake the jar and drink quickly as it thickens really fast.  Takes three times daily.

\*\*\*\*\*\*\*\*\*\*\*\*\*\*\*\*\*\*\*\*\*\*\*\*\*\*\*\*\*\*\*\*\*\*\*\*\*\*\*\*\*\*\*\*\*\*\*\*

## THERAPY CONSIDERATIONS:

- Fever bath three times weekly
- Salt Glow once daily.
- Steam bath twice weekly.
- Warm clay bath once weekly.

Apply charcoal, clay poultice or castor oil pack over breast nightly.  Also, you can place herbal tea mixture (leaves) on gauge and use as poultice.  Alternate or utilize poultices based on desired results.

\*\*\*\*\*\*\*\*\*\*\*\*\*\*\*\*\*\*\*\*\*\*\*\*\*\*\*\*\*\*\*\*\*\*\*\*\*\*\*\*\*\*\*\*\*\*\*\*\*\*\*\*

## STEAM BATH

The purpose of this therapy is to raise the body temperature and cause perspiration, which is a cleansing.

## ARTICLES NEEDED

* Bath mat     *Wooden chair     *Washcloth
*Electric Steam Kettle/Pot    *Two Basins ( Foot & Head)
*Glass of water    *Thermometer
*Hand Towel     *Steam Cabinet  or Shower Liner
*Large Bath Towel (To cover chair)

**PROCEDURES**  *(Duration of Therapy:  20-30 minutes)*
- Under chair, preheat electrical steam kettle before sitting under steam tent.  Ensure tent is draped on the floor so steam will not escape.
- Always pray before starting therapy.
- Place feet in foot basin with hot water throughout therapy.
- Basin for head, fill with ice water, wet wash cloth and place on forehead or top of head   Dip in water often to keep the head cool. (prevents  the brain from getting too hot)
- Take  temperature at beginning of therapy, then every 5 minutes; also  give  person  water  to drink as needed.
- Try to get  temperature up to at least 101, if possible.
- Upon completion, take a cold shower to cool the  body down quickly.  Turn around in  shower and   expose the whole body to the cold water.
- After cold shower, rest in bed, covered with sheet and blanket and out of all drafts for at least 30 minutes.

**CAUTION:  Use extreme caution with elderly and high blood pressure individuals.**

\*\*\*\*\*\*\*\*\*\*\*\*\*\*\*\*\*\*\*\*\*\*\*\*\*\*\*\*\*\*\*\*\*\*\*\*\*\*\*\*\*\*\*\*\*\*\*\*\*\*\*\*\*\*\*\*\*\*

# FEVER BATH
*(Increases White Blood Cells)*
For this therapy, assistance is needed.

## ARTICLES NEEDED

* Epsom salt
* Eucalyptus Oil (opt.)
* Pitcher or Container
* Glass of cool water with straw

* 2 Large Towels
* 2 Wash Cloths
* Ice Bags

## PROCEDURE

Make a note of the starting body temperature **before** bath. Place a large towel at bottom of tub; fill tub up with hot water; add 2 pounds of Epsom salt and 10 drops of eucalyptus oil (opt.). Assist person into tub. Ensure water is covering body; place another towel over breast area. Pour water over area with pitcher/ container. Induce fever to between 102 and 104 degrees. Add more hot water to tub as needed. Keep the head cool with washcloth and base of the neck **cool** with cold compresses. Drink copious quantity of cool water to compensate for sweating and to assist in cleansing. Treatment should last 20-30 minutes. End the bath with a brief cool shower to bring body temperature to normal (~98.6). Rest in bed thirty to sixty minutes.

Treatment should be carried out for two to four weeks, depending on the strength and energy of the individual.

## PRECAUTIONS

• Have bathroom warm.
• Ensure hot water does not scald person.
• Monitor person carefully.

If person feels faint, discontinue therapy and cool the body down.

\*\*\*\*\*\*\*\*\*\*\*\*\*\*\*\*\*\*\*\*\*\*\*\*\*\*\*\*\*\*\*\*\*\*\*\*\*\*\*\*\*\*\*\*\*\*\*\*\*\*\*\*

# THE SALT GLOW

The salt glow is a vigorous circulatory stimulate, and therefore a valuable tonic measure. As the name implies, salt is used with friction to make the skin flow with a fresh supply of blood. The particles of dead skin are removed, and after a sweating treatment, the pores are cleansed, leaving the skin soft, smooth, and glowing.

The degree of friction used is determined by the sensitivity of the individual's skin. You may wish to enjoy or perform a salt glow for an exhilarating and invigorating effect and preferably done in the bathtub or shower. The tonic effect may be increased by a hot and cold shower.

**ARTICLES NEEDED**
- Pan containing about two pounds of Epsom or coarse salt
- Towel

**PROCEDURE**
- Moisten salt with warm water
- Apply salt with both hands, spreading it over the skin and rubbing briskly towards the heart with back and forth movements.
- Proceed with each part of the body as follows:
  - Right arm
  - Left arm
  - Right leg

- Left leg
- Front and back of trunk (simultaneously)
- Sides of trunk and hips
- Hips
- Follow up with a hot then cold shower.
- Dry with a towel by brisk rubbing

**PRECAUTIONS**
- Have salt just moist enough (snow consistency) to cling to skin when applied. (If too wet, it will not produce the friction desired.
- Have room warm and work quickly to avoid chilling.

**GOOD FOR:**

| | |
|---|---|
| * Chronic Indigestion | * Diabetes |
| * Sluggish Circulation | * Low Blood Pressure |
| * Frequent Colds | *Weakness & Low Endurance |

*************************************************

**Enemas/Colonics** – Use warm bottled water, add 1 cup of fresh garlic (3 cloves) in 1 cup of water blended and strained. **(Perform when needed to relieve bowels of gas or constipation)**

*************************************************

# CHARCOAL

Charcoal is plain black wood which has been pulverized into powder. It's one of nature's finest magnetic sponges for absorbing toxins, poisons, pollutants, bacteria, pain from burns, just to name a few. When used internally, it is the most valuable single agent currently available for treating: drug overdose, poisoning, stomach distress, intestinal gas, toxic condition, vomiting. It may be used without side effects or overdose. It has no additives, chemicals, binders, etc.

**CHARCOAL POULTICE**:*(Use for: Inflammation, Boils, Tumors)* Make the poultice the size to meet your need. All you want to do is to cover the area needed. The paste is made by mixing equal parts of flaxseeds (either whole or ground) with the charcoal powder boiling water make a moderately thick paste but thin enough to spread thinly.

Spread the paste evenly over a paper tower or porous cloth cut to the proper size. Cover it with a top piece of towel the same size. Place this over the area to be treated and cover with a larger piece of household plastic. Now use a cloth or towel to cover and hold the poultice and plastic in place. Secure by stretch bandage or pin or tape. It can be messy.

Apply poultice immediately for 1-2 hours or a bedtime, leaving overnight. Absorption takes place almost immediately. Change poultice after each use. Wash or gently cleanse area when finished with cool water. Repeat as needed.

**CAUTION:** Charcoal is a powerful absorbent and will certainly absorb other drugs that one may be taking by prescription. Do not take charcoal with prescribe drugs. It will absorb penicillin, heart medicines, etc.

**************************************************

## OTHER POULTICES

**<u>Clay Poultice:</u>** Place on spots on the breast and leave on overnight.

**<u>Castor Oil Poultice</u>**:  Warm oil and saturate cloth and place area nightly.

\*\*\*\*\*\*\*\*\*\*\*\*\*\*\*\*\*\*\*\*\*\*\*\*\*\*\*\*\*\*\*\*\*\*\*\*\*\*\*\*\*\*\*\*

## PAIN SALVE

- 4 tbsp.  cayenne pepper (90 I.U. heat unit or
- higher)
- 1 tbsp.  peppermint oil
- ½ cup olive oil or coconut oil

*In glass jar, place all the ingredients; mix, and rub over area.*

**Caution:**  Do not rub eyes with hand, unless washed, after applying salve.

***Continue on this program until the Great Physician has His way!***

*MAY GOD RICHLY BLESS YOU AS YOU STRIVE TO MAKE LIFESTYLE CHANGES AND REACH A HIGHER LEVEL OF WHOLENESS:  PHYSICALLY, MENTALLY, AND SPIRITUALLY.*

# *Glossary*

This list of medical and non-medical terms is selected primarily from the pages of this book. Words defined here may include those occurring in more than one chapter, those key to understanding the material in a chapter, and those that may help clarify some of the definitions themselves.

**Axillary:** Located in the armpit.

**Benign:** Non-cancerous; a benign tumor means there is no cancer present.

**Biological therapy (immunotherapy):** A type of breast cancer treatment that boosts the body's immune system and increases its ability to fight cancer.

**Biopsy:** Diagnostic procedure that involves removing a small sample of suspicious tissue to determine whether or not it is cancerous; a suspicious breast lump will be biopsied to look for cancer cells.

**BRCA1 and BRCA2:** The two genes that, when mutated, are the cause of most inherited forms of breast and ovarian cancers.

**Breast:** The anterior or front region of the chest. The mammary gland.

**Carcinoma:** Type of cancer that originates in the cells that form the lining of a gland or organ.

**Chemotherapy:** Type of cancer treatment that involves destroy cancer cells. It's often used in conjunction with other forms of breast cancer treatment.

**Cyst:** A lump that's made of a small, fluid-filled sac.

**Detoxify:** To remove or neutralize the harmful activity of a toxic substance in the body.

**Disease:** A definite pathological process having a characteristic set of signs and symptoms. It may affect the whole body or any of its parts, and its prognosis may be known or unknown.

**Drug:** Medical meaning. Any chemical agent or medicinal substance (compound, preparation, remedy, etc.) used to promote health or to treat disease by causing a desired change within the body or on its surface. Popular meaning: Certain chemical compounds and plant substances that alter mood or mental or emotional state; some of these drugs are addicting.

**Duct:** Tubes located in the breast that allow milk to reach the nipple for breastfeeding.

**Ductal carcinoma in situ (DCIS):** Breast cancer that is confined to the milk ducts in the breast.

**Estrogen:** The hormone produced by the ovaries that gives women characteristics of the female sex. Estrogen is thought to encourage breast cancer cell growth.

**Estrogen receptor test:** A diagnostic laboratory test used to determine if a breast cancer is using estrogen to grow and if hormone therapy should be the treatment course.

**Fat Necrosis:** Uncommon but may be the basis for confusing and misdiagnosis of breast cancer. Trauma is presumed to be the cause, based on some type injury to the breasts. A sensitive mass often develops.

**Fibroadenoma:** A benign, unusually unilateral, firm, and nontender tumor of glandular and fibrous tissue.

**Fibrocystic:** It has been said to be the most common disorders of the breasts. The chief feature is the formation and growth of tiny cysts . Most women complain of tenderness and dull heaviness in both breasts. Rapid appearance and disappearance of the cysts is common in this condition.

**Hormone:** A chemical substance made in an endocrine gland and secreted into the bloodstream. The hormone then acts on some distant target within the body.
 **Hormone therapy (hormonal therapy):** Breast cancer treatment that uses hormones to either promote or inhibit the effects of certain hormones on the cancerous tissue.

**Infection:** (1) Invasion of the body, or one of its parts, by a harmful microorganism. (2) The disease thus caused by the invasion.

**Inflammation:** The body's four-alarm response to injury or infection; (1) pain (2) heat (3) reddening and (4) swelling. These local reactions signify that the body is rallying its forces to limit and repair the damage. Inflammation is thus not the same as infection, although the latter often triggers inflammation.

**Lifestyle:** The pattern of daily living that an individual develops.

**Localized cancer:** Cancer confined to one area (in this case, the breast) that hasn't spread elsewhere in the body.

**Lumpectomy: <u>Breast cancer surgery</u>** to remove the breast cancer lump and some surrounding tissue rather than the entire breast.

**Lymph nodes:** Small solid organs in the body that help to protect against foreign substances in the body. Breast cancer that has affected the lymph nodes may mean that the cancer has spread elsewhere in the body beyond the breast.

**Magnetic resonance imaging (MRI):** Diagnostic imaging test that provides three-dimensional views of the breast and any abnormalities.

**Malignant:** Cancerous, as in a malignant tumor.

**Mammography:** Diagnostic screening technique using X-ray images to check the breasts.

**Mastectomy:** The surgical removal of a breast; in a double mastectomy, both breasts are removed.

**Mastitis:** Inflammation of the breast, usually due to bacterial infection.

**Medical:** Pertaining to medicine, an evaluative process applied to the quality of clinical practice, often by peer review of routine or specially collected records of individual cases.

**Menopause:** The span of time during which the menstrual cycle wanes and gradually stops; also called change of life. It is the period when ovaries stop functioning and therefore menstruation and childbearing cease.

**Metastasize:** The spread of cancer beyond its initial site; if breast cancer has metastasized, it has spread beyond the breasts to other parts of the body.

**Microcalcifications:** Small calcium deposits formed in the breast tissue.

**Needle biopsy:** Diagnostic test using a needle to draw a tissue sample. The sample is used to test for cancer.

**Oncologist:** Medical professional who specializes in cancer (oncology).

**Pregnancy:** Being with child; the condition from conception to the expulsion of the fetus.

**Puberty:** The period during which secondary sexual characteristics develop and the reproductive organs become functional.

**Raloxifene:** Hormonal therapy drug that is used to help reduce breast cancer risk.

**Radiation therapy:** Type of cancer treatment that uses high doses of radiation (X-rays).

**Remission:** Term used when no signs of cancer are apparent after treatment.

**Stage:** Breast cancer is staged from 0 to IV, according to how large a tumor is and how advanced the cancer is — if and how far it has spread throughout the body. The lower the stage, the less advanced the breast cancer.

**Symptom:** What a person complains of – from palpitations to pain. A symptom is your body's signal to you that something is wrong (e.g., abdominal pain).

**Syndrome:** A group of signs or symptoms typical of a distinctive disease, which frequently occur together and form a distinctive clinical picture.

**Systemic therapy:** Breast cancer treatment that affects the entire body, such as chemotherapy.

**Tamoxifen:** Hormonal treatment in pill form used to treat breast cancer that is sensitive to estrogen. It's also used as a preventive therapy in women who have many risk factors for developing breast cancer.

**Therapy:** Any form of medical treatment.

**TNM system:** Classification of breast cancer based on three assessments — T for tumor size, N for lymph node involvement, and M for presence or absence of metastatic spread. The TMN classification aids in staging the cancer for making treatment decisions.

**Toxic:** Poisonous. Effect ranging from harmful to lethal, depending on the amount and the resistance of the individual.

**Tumor:** An abnormal mass that can be benign or malignant.

**Ultrasonography:** Diagnostic test for breast cancer that uses very high-frequency sound waves to help spot a tumor or breast abnormality. The sound waves are converted into a video or photo, which can indicate a tumor.

**Xeloda:** Brand name of the oral chemotherapy drug capecitabine, a hormonal therapy treatment for advanced breast cancer.

*About The Author*

Speaking of health, Patricia Sheffield, known as Sister Pat, is a servant of the Lord as a medical missionary with H.M.E.C. (Hope and Mercy Educational Center). H.M.E.C. is a *City Mission* dedicated to promoting faith in God, teaching the world about the soon coming Saviour, and proclaiming mankind's right to physical, mental and spiritual healing through Health Reform.

All of Sister Pat's credentials are "heaven approved." While a student of the Great Physician — Christ Jesus, she has sat at His feet since 1999, in an intense study of health and the gospel, according to the word of God. As a faithful ambassador of health, Sis Pat showcases the exalted pre-eminence of Biblical health principles, taught in the word of God, along with the system of healing ordained by heaven, making it the head and not the tail of true medical science.

When it comes to women's health, Sister Pat has an extreme passion for the complete, comprehensive care of women–from the womb to menopause and beyond. This is fulfilled in several areas of her ministry, such as Medical Missionary training, Pregnancy, Childbirth, & Midwifery education and services; health lecturers, personal consultations; therapeutic services; publications, and more. On the whole, her ministry is female specific— but male friendly.

Overall, Christ's commission in Matthew 28:18-20 is Sister Pat's Mission. Her travels, domestically and internationally, include several cities in the United States, London, Ghana, Zimbabwe, Malawi, Dominica, South Africa, Mozambique, Guatemala, Puerto Rico, Belize—just to highlight a few.

Giving all the glory, praises, and thanks to God, Sister Pat is ever grateful for the many healing blessings manifested in the lives she has been called to serve.

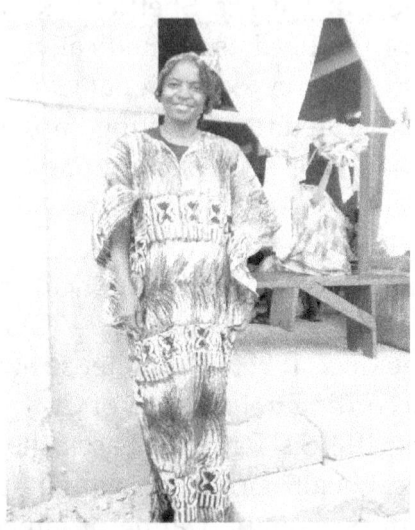

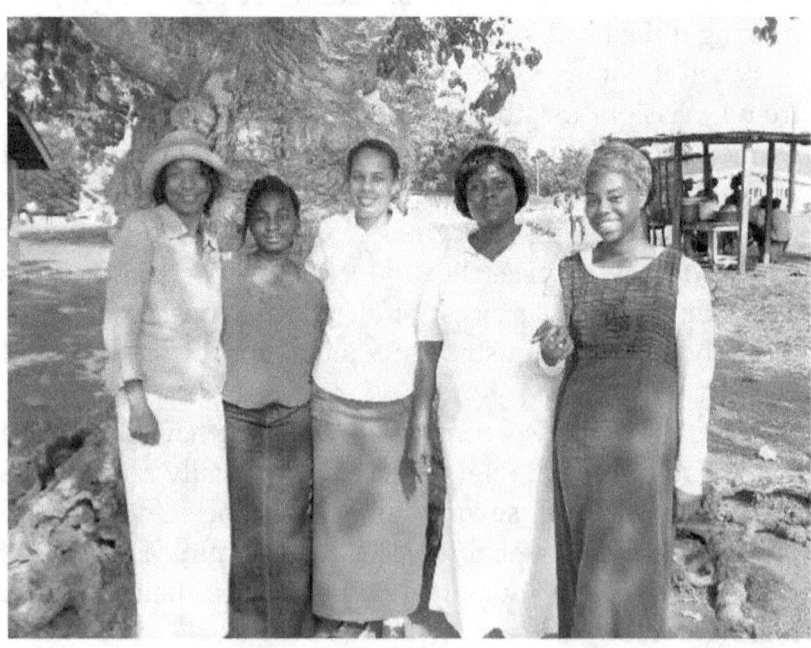

# The "Write" Things

This space serves as a convenient place to record breast notes, questions, answers, instructions, suggestions and anything of importance, that might be forgotten, unless noted when they occur to you.

Date_____

Question:_____

_____

_____

_____

Suggestions/Instructions/
Notes:_____

_____

_____

_____

_____

Date_____

Question:_____

_____

_____

_____

Suggestions/Instructions/
Notes:_____

_____

_____

_____

_____

Date_____

Question:_____

_____

_____

_____

Suggestions/Instructions/
Notes:_____

_____

_____

_____

Date_____

Question:_____

_____

_____

_____

Suggestions/Instructions/
Notes:_____

_____

_____

_____

_____

Date_____

Question:_____

_____

_____

_____

Suggestions/Instructions/
Notes:_____

_____

_____

_____

_____

Date_____

Question:_____

_____

_____

_____

Suggestions/Instructions/
Notes:_____

_____

_____

_____

_____

Date_____

Question:_____

_____

_____

_____

Suggestions/Instructions/
Notes:_____

_____

_____

_____

_____

Date_____

Question:_____

_____

_____

_____

Suggestions/Instructions/
Notes:_____

_____

_____

_____

Date_____

Question:_____

_____

_____

_____

Suggestions/Instructions/
Notes:_____

_____

_____

_____

_____

Date_____

Question:_____

_____

_____

_____

Suggestions/Instructions/
Notes:_____

_____

_____

_____

_____

Date_____

Question:_____

_____

_____

_____

Suggestions/Instructions/
Notes:_____

_____

_____

_____

_____

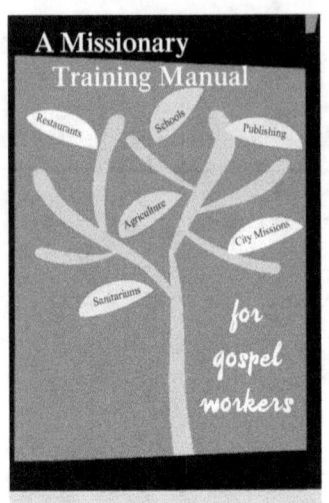

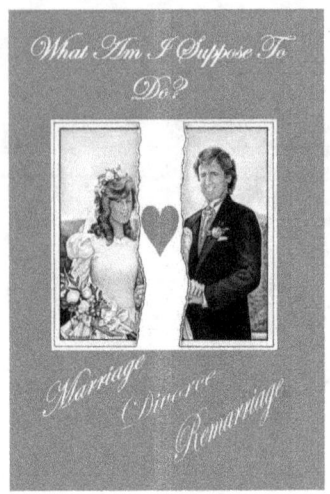

## Hope and Mercy Educational Center
# Book Gallery

*Educational publications covering many subjects. Books that contain more than words....LIFE. They are full of principles, with practical messages.*

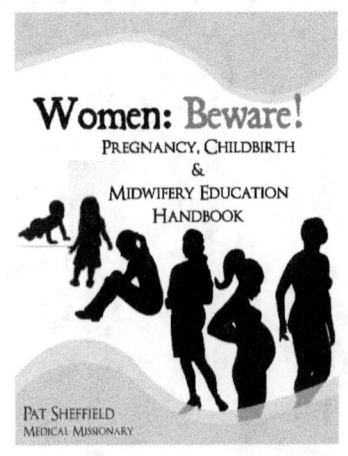

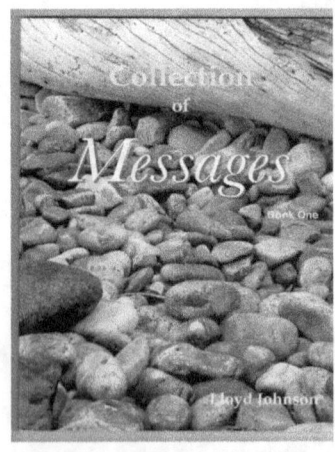

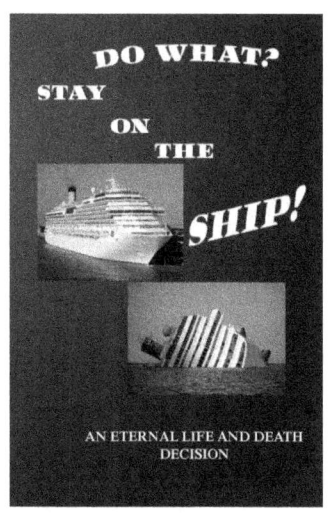

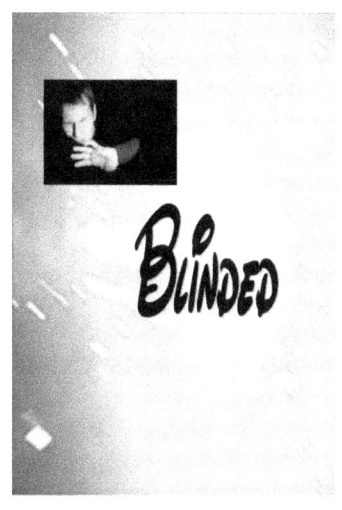

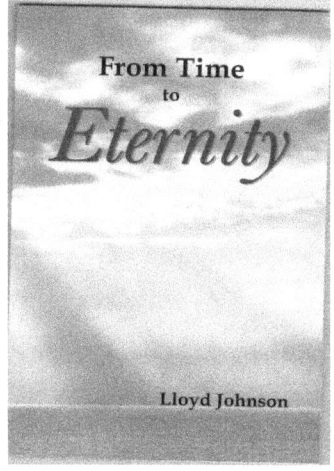

Order these books directly from H.M.E.C. or online** at www.amazon.com.

Discount prices for orders of 50 or more books via H.M.E.C.

** *Except 'From Time to Eternity" and "Collection of Messages"*

We would love to send you a catalog of titles we publish or even hear your thoughts, reactions, suggestions, criticism, about things in our publications.

Just write or call us at:

**H.M.E.C.**
**(Hope and Mercy Educational Center)**
*A City Mission*
2827 Hwy 70 West
Camden, Tennessee   38320
(731) 584-7004

hmecschool@yahoo.com

# SEEKING TRUE EDUCATION?
## ........LOOK NO FURTHER!!

### *"AN OUTPOST CAMPUS"*

Hope and Mercy Educational Center (H.M.E.C.) Pattern School, a Christian institution focusing on the education, health and welfare of all ages to provide "true higher education".

H.M.E.C.'s goal is to educate, not only in a knowledge of the Scriptures, but give a practical training that fit students to go forth and give the gospel message to the world as self-supporting missionaries in the field to which they are called.

Every course is designed to lead students to Jesus and to enhance their ministry. Curriculum includes:

- **AGRICULTURE -** all phases of agriculture and farm mechanics

- **BIBLE -** Evangelism, Canvassing, Bible Studies, Prophecy, Sanctuary Message, Sacred History

- **COMMUNICATIONS -** Voice & Speech, Public Evangelism, Marketing, Sacred Music, Poetry

- **HEALTH -** Medical missionary work, Anatomy & Physiology, Midwifery and Childbirth Education (women only), Massage Therapy, Hydrotherapy, Natural Remedies, City Mission Activities

- **MANUAL LABOR -** Painting, Carpentry/Woodworking, Auto Mechanics, Electrical Mechanics, Welding, Masonry

- **PRACTICAL ARTS -** Printing, Bookkeeping, Arts/Crafts, Sewing, Cooking

- **INTERNSHIP/APPRENTICESHIP -** A concentrated and dedicated time to mature and develop skills in various industry lines and/or ministry environments i.e., Sanitarium, City Mission, Health Food Store, etc..

We welcome students (youth and seniors) to H.M.E.C. who would like to *demonstrate* their ability through their *willingness* to work, their *fidelity* to principle, and their *firmness* for truth!

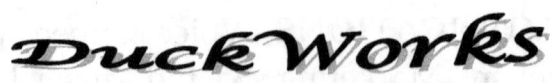

An Industry of H.M.E.C. School